S0-AEB-634

So you're having

Angioplasty

So you're having

Angioplasty

STEPHEN FORT MD
VICTORIA K. FOULGER RN

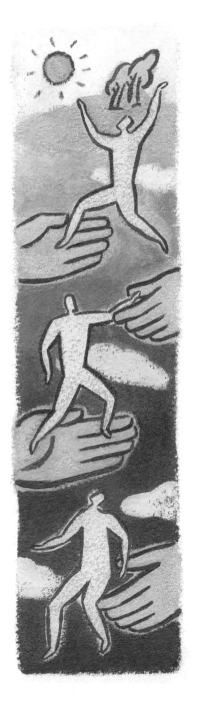

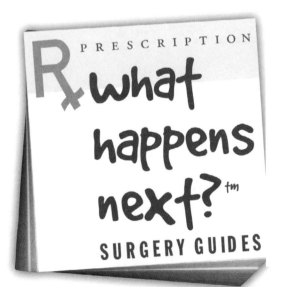

PRESCRIPTION

R what happens next?™

SURGERY GUIDES

SCRIPT
medical press inc.

First published in Canada in 2001 by
SCRIPT Medical Press, Inc.
Box 38096, 550 Eglinton Avenue West
Toronto, Ontario M5N 3A8
www.whathappensnext.ca

Copyright © SCRIPT Medical Press, Inc.

All rights reserved. No part of this book may be reproduced, stored in a retrival system, or transmitted in any form or by any means, electronic, mechanical, photocopying, recording, or otherwise without permission in writing from the publisher.

CANADIAN CATALOGUING IN PUBLICATION DATA

Fort, Stephen, 1960–
        So you're having angioplasty, what happens next?

(What happens next surgery guides)
Includes bibliographical reference and index.
ISBN 0-9688982-0-3

1. Angioplasty—Popular works. I. Foulger, Victoria, 1971–
II. Title. III. Series.

RD598.35.A53F66 2001   617.4'13   C2001–902344–8

General Editor: Helen Byrt
Book Design and Typesetting: Rocket Design
Cover Illustration: Ross Paul Lindo
Author Photographs: Doug Nicholson, Media Source
Book Illustrations: Bernie Freedman

Publishing Consultant: Malcolm Lester & Associates

Photographs on pages 56, 59, 128 courtesy of JOMED Canada Inc.; photographs on pages 65 and 129 courtesy of Guidant Corporation; photographs on pages 65, 130, 131 courtesy of Boston Scientific Corporation; photograph on page 66 courtesy of EndiCOR Medical, Inc.; photograph on page 131 courtesy of Medtronic, Inc.; and photograph on page 14 courtesy of Media Source. Rotablator® is a registered trademark of Boston Scientific Corporation or its affiliates; Cutting Balloon™ is a trademark of IVT, Inc.; FilterWire™ is trademark of Embolic Protection, Inc.

The publisher has made every effort to obtain permissions for use of copyrighted material in this book; any errors or omissions will be corrected in the next printing.

Printed and bound in Canada
01 02 03 04 5 4 3 2 1

To Alexander Kai,
and our parents

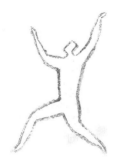

[FORTHCOMING BOOKS *in the* SERIES]

So You're Having
Heart Bypass Surgery
—What Happens Next?

So You're Having
Prostate Surgery
—What Happens Next?

So You're Having
Gall Bladder Surgery
—What Happens Next?

acknowledgments

W E HAVE MANY PEOPLE TO THANK FOR LAUNCHING US
with their enthusiasm and keeping us fueled with
their time.
The publisher would like to thank Martin Anstice and Joy
Macdonald for early inspiration and Dr. Charlie Lazzam,
Judy Hemming and Karen Mackie for early input (and
laughing at our first title). Murray Maynard and Joel
Rochon of JOMED Canada, Eli Lilly Canada, Dana
Andrea, and Dr. Stuart McCluskey helped the concept
become reality, and Hans Aarden supplied his unique
brand of creative enthusiasm. Bernie Freedman gave us
devotion well beyond the call of duty, as did our publishing
team: Jenny Lass, Malcolm Lester, Andrea Knight, Brian
Cartwright, Carol Thomas, Dorothy Lyszkiewicz, Megan
Morrison: thank you.

The authors' thanks go to Celina Ainsworth and Kathy
Camelon for expert assistance with the self-help chapter.

Finally, we acknowledge with gratitude the patients and
families who so willingly shared their experiences with us:
Arni Cohn, the late Robert (Bobby) Frew, Mrs. Joyce Frew,
Bill Hogarth, and Dr. T. Hofmann.

disclaimer

THE INFORMATION PROVIDED IN THIS BOOK MAY NOT apply to all patients, all clinical situations, all hospitals, or all eventualities, and is not intended to be a substitute for the advice of a qualified physician or other medical professional. Always consult a qualified physician about anything that affects your health, especially before starting an exercise program or using a complementary therapy not prescribed by your doctor.

The financial support received from the sponsors of this book does not constitute an endorsement by the authors or publisher of the sponsors or their products. Similarly, the naming of any organization, product or therapy in this book does not imply endorsement by the authors or publisher and the omission of any such names does not indicate disapproval by the authors or publisher.

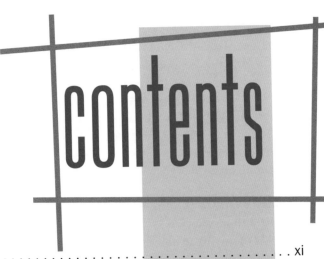

contents

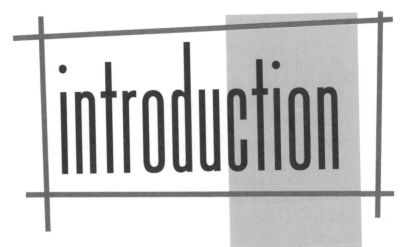

introduction

I F YOU HAVE BEEN DIAGNOSED WITH CARDIOVASCULAR DISEASE, you are not alone. It is estimated that one in four Canadians—around 8 million people—has some form of cardiovascular disease. Around 40,000 people have a heart attack each year in Canada and cardiovascular disease is now Canada's number one cause of death. The most recent figures show that 36 percent of all male deaths and 39 percent of all female deaths were due to cardiovascular disease.

So what happens next?

There are many treatments for cardiovascular disease, including drug therapy, lifestyle changes, angioplasty, and coronary artery bypass surgery (a "heart bypass"). The aim of this book is to take you through the angioplasty procedure, step-by-step. At every stage, from diagnosis to recovery, you will know what your options are and what to expect.

Coronary angioplasty, or **percutaneous transluminal coronary angioplasty (PTCA)** to give it its proper title, is an excellent treatment option for most patients with angina and is also becoming increasingly important in the treatment of acute heart attacks. It does not refer to a single operation on your blood vessel, but to many different types of techniques that involve placing a tube (or catheter) in your artery to improve the blood flow. Some techniques are more suitable to treat certain blockages than others, and some are more successful than others. In this book you will find several chapters covering all the devices and techniques available to your physician. Our aim is not to make you nervous, but to help you understand why a particular technique is—or is not—being used in your case.

To complete the picture, Chapter 3 will help you decide whether angioplasty is right for you and Chapter 11 will help you to decide whether your angioplasty has been successful.

Just as a combination of factors contributed to your heart disease, a combination of treatments is the most effective way to treat it. As clinicians, we are only too aware that no medical intervention can work by itself. A healthy diet, regular exercise, smoking cessation, and complementary therapies also have a part to play in enabling you to take control of your heart disease. Self-help shouldn't just be an afterthought: it is the core of your treatment, so we have devoted a substantial chapter to strategies that you can use to help yourself (Chapter 10).

This book is not designed to replace consultation with your cardiologist or cardiac surgeon, but to add to it. Our goal is to provide you, your family, and your friends with enough information to understand what your physician is recommending to you, and why. We hope that this book will help you to ask the right questions, and more fully understand the answers and recommendations that he or she gives you.

You are in charge of your health, and never more so than with cardiovascular disease. Your physician can advise and treat you, but the health of your heart is, ultimately, in your hands. Only you can decide which treatment to have, and only you can make the lifestyle changes that will put you on a road to better health. We hope that this book will equip you with the knowledge to make the decisions that are right for you.

Good luck!

coronary artery disease and you

What Happens in this Chapter

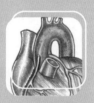

- The facts on coronary artery disease
- The likely reasons you have clogged arteries
- The symptoms of angina and a heart attack
- How you can take control of your future

*Your heart is a pump the size of your fist. It beats about 60 times a minute to keep blood circulating through your body, carrying nutrients and oxygen to your tissues. It is made of a unique type of muscle called **myocardium**—the only muscle in the body that keeps contracting without needing a break. The blood supply that allows the myocardium to do this comes from the coronary arteries. When the coronary arteries get blocked by disease, the blood supply to the myocardium is interrupted, resulting in angina or a heart attack. The aim of angioplasty is to clear the blockage and restore normal blood flow to the myocardium.*

How the Heart Works

THE HUMAN HEART IS AN AMAZING PIECE OF ENGINEERING. It is actually two pumps in one: the right half of the heart pumps blood to the lungs to pick up oxygen, while the left half receives the oxygen-rich blood from the lungs and pumps it onwards, around the rest of the body. Valves inside the heart keep the blood moving in the right direction and a thin, lubricated membrane outside (called the **pericardium**) ensures that the pumping heart can move easily.

The heart muscle itself (the myocardium) needs a good blood supply to keep contracting, especially during exercise or exertion. The arteries that supply the heart muscle with blood are called the **coronary arteries**—so-called because from above they look like a crown. The coronary arteries branch off the **aorta** (the main blood vessel in your body) at the point where the oxygen-rich blood leaves the heart, so the heart muscle is the first organ in your body to receive oxygenated blood.

Coronary Artery Disease

Coronary artery disease is a condition in which one or more of the coronary arteries becomes narrowed, so that the heart muscle does not receive enough oxygen. Both angina and heart attacks are usually caused by coronary artery disease, which is the leading cause of death in developed countries.

Coronary artery disease is a form of **atherosclerosis**—a process where the arteries gradually clog up like old water pipes (see More Detail box). Over several decades, cholesterol, calcium, and other substances build up under the artery's inner lining, creating a blockage that starts to restrict the flow of blood down the artery (see Figure 1). The technical term for this blockage is a **plaque.**

Figure 1. How a Plaque Develops

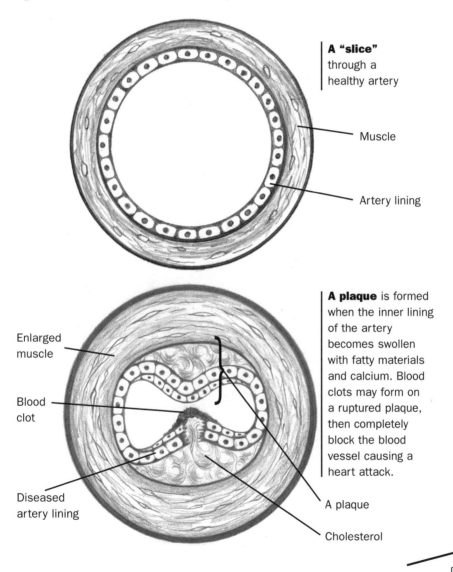

A "slice" through a healthy artery

Muscle

Artery lining

Enlarged muscle

Blood clot

Diseased artery lining

A plaque is formed when the inner lining of the artery becomes swollen with fatty materials and calcium. Blood clots may form on a ruptured plaque, then completely block the blood vessel causing a heart attack.

A plaque

Cholesterol

> "We were staying in a hotel and my husband went to a meeting, so I was alone, and suddenly, as I was walking on the beach, I got very, very bad angina. Somehow I made it back to my chair and waited for my husband. I knew something had happened...I was so weak."
>
> **Mrs. C.V.**

Plaques can become surprisingly large before they start to restrict blood flow because, at first, the artery does its best to compensate for the blockage by stretching and expanding its outer wall. However, this so-called "positive remodeling" has its limits, and gradually the inside of the artery becomes so narrowed that blood flow is reduced, and the symptoms of angina start to appear.

Atherosclerosis
— What's in a Name?

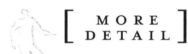

[MORE DETAIL]

Coronary artery disease is caused by a process called atherosclerosis. This strange-sounding name comes from the Greek words for "hard" (sclerosis) and "oatmeal" (athero) because this is what atherosclerosis looked like to the first doctors—a hard, lumpy, fat-filled coating on the insides of arteries.

Atherosclerosis can occur in any blood vessel in the body. In coronary arteries, the blockages cause angina or heart attacks. In the brain, they cause strokes. In the legs, they can cause poor circulation (claudication and gangrene).

Why Do You Have Coronary Artery Disease?

It is still not clear what triggers coronary artery disease, despite many years of research. It can start as early as the teenage years: post-mortem studies on young soldiers who died during the Vietnam War showed that they had early signs of atherosclerosis. It is clear, however, that there are a number of factors that increase people's chances of getting coronary artery disease—so-called **cardiac risk factors.** These include lifestyle choices such as smoking and lack of exercise, as well as "unmodifiable" risk factors, such as a family history of heart disease (see Key Point box).

The good news is that if you change the risk factors in your life you can improve your future health considerably, even if you already have coronary artery disease.

$$\left[\begin{array}{c} \text{K E Y} \\ \text{P O I N T} \end{array} \right]$$

Major risk factors for coronary artery disease

Nothing is certain in life, but if you have one or more of these risk factors, then you are more likely to develop coronary artery disease. The more severe the risk factor, the more severe your coronary artery disease is likely to be.

- Family history
- Hyperlipidemia (e.g., high blood cholesterol)
- Smoking
- Diabetes
- High blood pressure
- Obesity
- Sedentary lifestyle

Angina

Usually, the first sign of coronary artery disease is **angina**, a chest pain that starts during exercise and gets better during rest. Most commonly, angina feels like a dull, heavy, constricting sensation that starts in the center of the chest and may spread into the throat or down one arm.

Angina happens when there is an inadequate supply of blood to the myocardium. The heart muscle becomes starved of oxygen and toxins build up, causing cramp-like pain. It is also called **myocardial ischemia**—literally, a reduction of blood to the heart muscle. Angina usually appears first during physical exercise or emotional stress because the heart is beating faster and more strongly, and requires more oxygen.

Figure 2. The Coronary Arteries

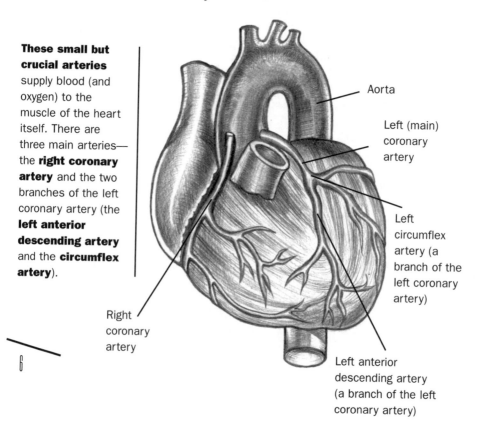

These small but crucial arteries supply blood (and oxygen) to the muscle of the heart itself. There are three main arteries— the **right coronary artery** and the two branches of the left coronary artery (the **left anterior descending artery** and the **circumflex artery**).

Aorta

Left (main) coronary artery

Left circumflex artery (a branch of the left coronary artery)

Right coronary artery

Left anterior descending artery (a branch of the left coronary artery)

If the blockages in the coronary arteries become severe, angina may be experienced even when resting. This is called **unstable angina**, and is a serious condition: a small number of patients who develop this form of severe angina are likely to have a heart attack within the next few weeks or months.

Not everyone feels pain with angina. "Painless" angina (also known as **silent ischemia**) can show up on an electrocardiogram (ECG), although the patient may be unaware of it or experience it as a non-painful symptom such as breathlessness. Silent ischemia is more common than was previously thought, and it may be due to shorter, or less severe, episodes of ischemia than those causing typical angina symptoms. Silent ischemia is treated in the same way as typical angina.

Although angina is most commonly caused by coronary artery disease, it can occasionally result from other heart conditions, for instance a disease of the heart valve called **aortic stenosis** (see Glossary).

A Heart Attack

In angina, blood still flows down the coronary artery and some oxygen reaches the heart muscle. By contrast, in a heart attack (or **myocardial infarction**), the coronary artery is blocked very suddenly and completely, causing a small area of muscle to die and a scar to form. The symptoms of a heart attack are usually different from the symptoms of angina (see Key Point box).

Many heart attacks occur in people with

"Back in 1965 we didn't even know there was such a thing as angina. I think my Mum had it, but they all thought 'pleurisy'— nobody spoke about angina. Father had a coronary thrombosis, too, so it does run in the family."

Robert (Bobby) Frew

> "When I had my heart attack it was the first indication of any heart problem. I had some shortness of breath, but never made the connection."
>
> **Arni Cohn**

no previous warning signs of angina. In addition, up to one quarter of heart attacks are "silent," without any chest pain. The cause of such silent heart attacks is currently unknown. However, since they are more common in people with diabetes—who often have damaged nerves—one theory is that silent heart attacks may result from abnormalities in the nerves that supply the heart, so people simply don't feel the pain.

Every chest pain is not angina or a heart attack. There can be many other reasons for chest pain, for instance, indigestion or pneumonia. Always see your physician if you experience pains in your chest.

[**KEY POINT**]

If you have the following symptoms you are more likely to be having a heart attack than angina

- Severe, heavy, crushing pain in your chest
- Pain that lasts more than 20 to 30 minutes
- Pain that does not go away when you rest
- No relief from sublingual nitroglycerine
- Breathlessness
- Nausea and, sometimes, vomiting
- Fainting or lightheadedness
- Rapid heartbeat
- Pallor and sweating

If you think you are having a heart attack, dial 911 right away. Do not waste time calling your cardiologist or family doctor.

If you have coronary artery disease, it is likely that you also have atherosclerosis in other arteries of your body. This means that you are at greater risk of having a stroke (due to atherosclerosis in the brain) or poor circulation in other vital organs such as your kidneys. But don't despair. The future is in your hands. Remember, only one cardiac risk factor can't be altered—your family history. Everything else can be changed and it is never too early to start. For advice on what you can do to help yourself, see Chapter 10.

What Happens Next?

If your physician thinks you have angina, there are a number of ways to confirm that you have it, find out the reason for it, and decide how serious it is. You may be sent for "non-invasive" tests such as a **treadmill test**, a **nuclear perfusion scan**, or an **echocardiogram** (see Glossary for details of these tests), which will show how well your heart is working. You may then be sent for **coronary angiography**, an "invasive" test that involves placing a tube (catheter) into your body to see what state your coronary arteries

> "They told me I had 15 percent damage. I found it hard to accept that my heart won't regenerate, grow back like fingernails or skin, but you have to accept it. You have to look at what is behind you, what you want to do in front of you, and plan."
>
> **Arni Cohn**

are in. Coronary angiography is covered in the next chapter. Your physician may also prescribe lipid-lowering medication at this stage to slow down the progression of atherosclerosis throughout your body, ASA (Aspirin) to reduce the risk of having a heart attack, and anti-anginal drugs to relieve your angina symptoms.

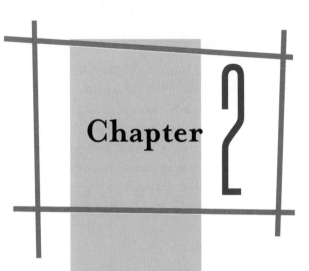

Chapter 2

coronary angiography

— YOUR HEART ON TV

What Happens in this Chapter

- Step-by-step guide to coronary angiography
- The risks and benefits
- Decoding your angiogram—and your diagnosis

Coronary angiography gives you and your medical team the inside story on your heart. It is not a treatment, but a diagnostic tool—a way of finding out exactly what is wrong with you. By injecting a special dye into the arteries of your heart and looking at the X-ray picture on a TV screen in real time, your physician can see which blood vessels are blocked, where, and how badly. This will help him or her to decide whether you need angioplasty, bypass surgery, or just drug therapy.

What is Coronary Angiography?

ANGIOGRAPHY SIMPLY MEANS TAKING PICTURES ("-graphy") of blood vessels ("angio-"). Coronary angiography thus means taking pictures of the blood vessels of the heart. The end result is an **angiogram**—an X-ray picture of your heart's own blood supply, and the most useful information that you and your medical team could have. Angiography is usually a separate procedure that takes place several days or weeks before you have your angioplasty, but an increasing number of people go on to have their angioplasty right after their angiography—so-called **ad-hoc angioplasty** (see page 20).

Blood vessels don't normally show up on X-rays, so an angiogram is created by injecting a dye that is visible to X-rays (radio-opaque) into the blood vessels of the heart. The physician then uses the X-ray machine to guide him or her through the procedure and record the pictures. There are three main coronary arteries that supply blood to the heart muscle (see Figure 2, page 6). During the angiogram your physician will look at all three of these arteries to check for disease. From the angiogram, your physician will be able to tell whether or not your coronary arteries are diseased, how badly, and which arteries are affected. If needed, the pumping action of your heart muscle can also be recorded—a procedure called a **left ventricular angiogram** (see page 17).

Angiography is an invaluable tool and a useful test to guide your treatment. However, as with all medical procedures, there are risks involved that you should be fully aware of before having your angiogram done (see More Detail box, page 22).

Help Yourself to Better Pictures

- It is normal to feel anxious, particularly if you are having a coronary angiogram for the first time. It may help to talk to someone else who has had the procedure. Your physician or nurse may be able to put you in touch with someone.

- Make a list of questions that you want to ask your doctor or nurse and take the list with you on the day of your procedure. If you do not understand something you have been told, ask for an explanation. Having a friend or family member with you can help. Do not sign the consent form if you are unhappy about anything.

- Try to ask everything you want to know before you go into the catheterization laboratory because once the procedure is underway, your medical team will be concentrating on the task at hand.

- Try not to move around to get a better view of the X-ray monitors because your heart will move, spoiling the pictures. The camera will be placed in the best possible position for quick and easy recording. If you can't see properly, ask your physician to show you the pictures at the end.

- If you feel any pain during the procedure, or experience any problems in your arm, leg, or chest afterwards, tell the medical team immediately.

Arrival in the Hospital

You will probably be one of a number of patients undergoing the same procedure that day. Although the angiography procedure only takes 20 to 30 minutes, you will probably be in the hospital for 6 to 8 hours in total.

While the exact arrangements vary from hospital to hospital, you are likely to be asked to follow these instructions en route to your angiogram:

- Don't eat or drink anything the morning of your procedure.

- Shave your groin before you go to the hospital, unless you have been told otherwise.

- Arrive at the hospital and report to the ward or admissions desk.

- Take your regular medication with a sip of water as you would do normally, unless told otherwise.

The clinic staff will then

- Carry out blood tests to check that your kidneys are working properly and that you are not anemic.

- Ask you to sign a consent form. At this point, the risks of your coronary angiogram procedure should be explained to you (see also More Detail box, page 22). If you do not understand something, now is the time to ask questions.

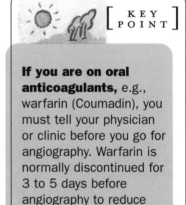

KEY POINT

If you are on oral anticoagulants, e.g., warfarin (Coumadin), you must tell your physician or clinic before you go for angiography. Warfarin is normally discontinued for 3 to 5 days before angiography to reduce the risk of heavy bleeding from the wound site.

The Cath Lab

When you reach the cardiac catheterization laboratory (or **cath lab**) you will be introduced to all the staff. In addition to your physician, there will be nurses and technicians, and, possibly, a junior physician. The staffing arrangements will vary from hospital to hospital. One of the first things you may notice is the temperature. The temperature inside modern cath labs is deliberately kept low to ensure reliable running of the X-ray and recording equipment. Since you will be wearing a thin gown, you may feel a little uncomfortable until you are settled on the X-ray table and covered in sterile drapes.

The table is narrow and not designed with comfort in mind, but try to make yourself as comfortable as possible. If you need another pillow, ask for one. Although a coronary angiogram is a relatively short procedure (under an hour, compared to an angioplasty that can sometimes take many hours) your comfort is important. Apart from the fact that cath lab staff want you to be happy, there is also a practical reason for making you comfortable: if you move around a lot it will be harder for the physician to get good pictures.

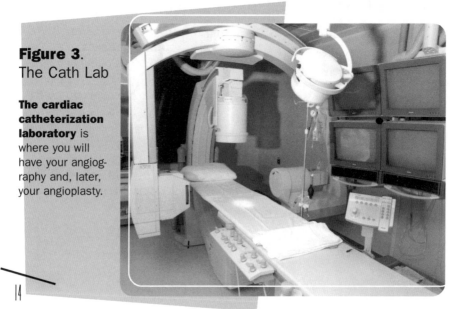

Figure 3.
The Cath Lab

The cardiac catheterization laboratory is where you will have your angiography and, later, your angioplasty.

Preparing for the Angiogram

Once you are lying on the X-ray table, the lab staff will attach leads to your chest and legs, just like when you had an electrocardiogram (ECG or EKG). These will allow your heart rate and rhythm to be monitored during the procedure.

The place on your skin where the tubes (or catheters) will be inserted will now be washed with a sterilizing solution to prevent infection. Since most sterilizing solutions contain alcohol, expect the fluid to feel cold. Most physicians use the groin to insert the catheters, although your physician may choose to use your arm (see page 61).

You will notice TV screens (monitors) on one side of you. This is where your X-ray pictures will be displayed during your procedure. You will be able to see some, but not all, of the pictures. The X-ray camera in front of your chest will sometimes block your view. Inform your physician if at any stage the X-ray camera comes too close for comfort.

The Angiography Procedure

Angiography uses a technique called **cardiac catheterization**, which means inserting one or more tubes into the heart. Although this sounds dramatic, it's actually a very simple concept because the tubes (or catheters) do not enter the heart through the chest wall, but through your blood vessels. Physicians quickly realized that since all blood vessels connect to the heart, it would be possible to insert a tube into the heart by feeding it into any blood vessel in the body. For angiography, the catheters are inserted into an artery in the arm

"I saw them take the tube out of my groin and I was amazed at how long it was, and the fact it gets all the way up to the heart."

Arni Cohn

or groin and are simply pushed along quite painlessly until they enter the heart—and the coronary arteries (see Figure 5, page 50). The dye can then be injected along the catheter into the coronary arteries.

The first step in coronary angiography is making the incision so that the catheters can enter an artery in your groin or arm. To make the incision more comfortable for you, the cath lab team will "freeze" your skin with an injection of local anesthetic. A small incision is then made into the skin by a scalpel, then a needle and a short tube called a **sheath** are inserted into your blood vessel. Even after the anesthetic, you may still feel some pulling and pushing in your groin, but it should not be painful.

Once the sheath is safely in place, your physician will insert the long catheters all the way to your heart. He or she will place the tips of the catheters in each of your three coronary arteries under X-ray guidance. Radio-opaque dye is then injected into your blood vessels. Any narrowings in the blood vessels will be displayed on the TV monitors, so the cath lab team can record the position and severity of the diseased areas. Because disease in blood vessels can sometimes affect just one part of the vessel wall without affecting the rest, your physician will need to see different views of your blood vessels. He or she will move the X-ray camera around and take pictures on both sides of your chest.

Because your heart moves with every breath you take, you will be asked to either hold your breath, or take a deep breath in and hold your breath, while the pictures are being taken.

The whole procedure takes only 20 to 30 minutes and most patients find it relatively easy to tolerate.

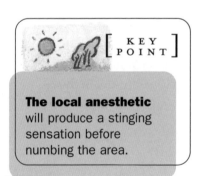

[KEY POINT]

The local anesthetic will produce a stinging sensation before numbing the area.

Left Ventricular Angiography

At the beginning or end of your angiogram procedure, another type of catheter, called a **pig tail catheter**, is often used to look at the muscular pumping action of the heart and the health of the heart valves. This is called a **left ventricular** (or **LV**) **angiogram**. When the dye is injected for the LV angiogram you may feel a peculiar warm sensation spreading around your body as the dye travels through your blood vessels. Another odd side effect is the feeling that you have passed urine. Do not worry, this is just an illusion and is entirely harmless.

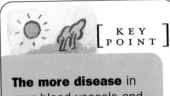

[**KEY POINT**]

The more disease in your blood vessels and the more blood vessels that are affected, the more likely you are to be recommended bypass surgery.

Sheath Removal and Bed Rest

Once the pictures have been taken, your physician will withdraw all the catheters. The sheath in your groin, through which the catheters were inserted, will usually be removed immediately afterwards. To reduce the risk of bleeding from the wound until the artery heals by forming a blood clot, one of the cath lab team members will either apply pressure manually (by pressing on your groin with his or her hands) or use a specially designed clamp-like device. Pressure, however applied, is usually needed for up to 30 minutes. To make sure that the blood vessel does not start to bleed again, you will be kept in bed for a few hours before being allowed to walk around. During this period, you and your puncture site will be closely supervised by a nurse.

In some hospitals, your blood vessel will be sealed using a special piece of equipment called a **closure device** (see page 60).

What Does Your Angiogram Mean?

"The main discomfort is that you can't move, especially afterwards, when, of course, you have to be immobile and your bladder is irritated from the dye. I didn't realize that I should have asked for a bedpan before the nurse put the press on me. I know it's a small thing, but at the time it was very uncomfortable."

Mrs. C.V.

"After my angiogram they told me I had a 90 percent blockage in the circumflex artery."

Mrs. C.V.

Once you have had your angiogram and are back in the ward or recovery area, you will probably be quite anxious to know the results. Sometimes your physician will tell you what he or she has seen while you are still in the cath lab. If this didn't happen, you will have to wait until your physician sees you shortly after your procedure. At this stage you should be looking for a full and clear explanation of your condition. Your physician will bring together the results of all your investigations, as well as your angiogram, to create a complete picture. He or she should be able to tell you exactly what is wrong, how serious your heart disease is, and what treatment will be best for you.

In general, mild disease (less than 50 percent narrowing) of one, two, or three of your blood vessels is usually treated with medication and diet. In moderate disease, where 50 to 70 percent of the artery is blocked, treatment depends on how bad your symptoms are and the results of other cardiac tests. Severe "single-vessel" disease (more than 70 percent narrowing of one blood vessel) is usually treated with angioplasty. Severe "three-vessel" disease is more likely to be treated with bypass surgery. For more on your treatment choices, see Chapter 3.

Figure 4. Coronary Angiograms

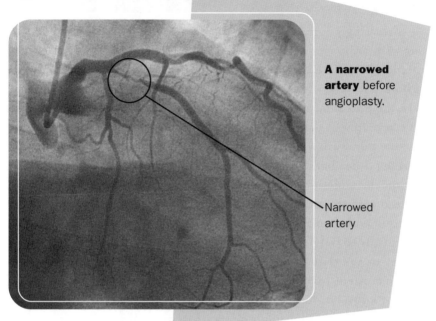

A narrowed artery before angioplasty.

Narrowed artery

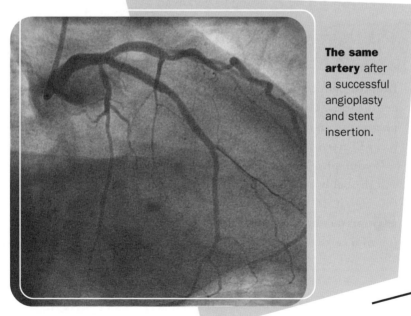

The same artery after a successful angioplasty and stent insertion.

Ad-Hoc Angioplasty

It is increasingly common for angioplasty to follow angiography in the same visit, although there is a lot of variation between hospitals. This procedure is called **ad-hoc, same-sitting,** or **carry-on angioplasty**. It has both potential advantages and disadvantages for you.

On the plus side, there is no need for a second hospital visit, you don't have to wait days or weeks for your angioplasty, and there is only one puncture wound in your groin or arm.

On the other hand, it is difficult to make decisions while you are lying on the table in the cath lab. You will need to decide whether to go ahead with the angioplasty right then, without any further chance to consult with family or another physician. You will not have the opportunity to weigh the pros and cons of angioplasty and bypass surgery, or the risks of the angioplasty procedure itself. When you sign the consent form before going into the cath lab, the physician does not know how bad your heart disease is and can only estimate the risks of your ad-hoc angioplasty procedure. If your disease turns out to be severe, you may want more time to think about the risks of angioplasty before agreeing to go ahead.

What Happens Next?

In most people, angiography gives clear answers and the next steps are obvious. However, you may need some further tests before your physician can decide which treatment is best for you. In this case, you will need to attend one or more further clinic appointments.

If your physician recommends angioplasty or bypass surgery, you will probably be referred to a specialist as a next step. The reason for this is that not all physicians who specialize in angiography perform angioplasty, and none of them performs bypass surgery: this is the job of a cardiac surgeon.

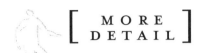

Single-, double-, or triple-vessel disease ⟿ Disease in one, two, or three of the coronary arteries (for more on coronary arteries, see Figure 2, page 6).

A plaque ⟿ The technical term for the blockage in your coronary artery. Plaques are made of cholesterol, scar tissue, and, sometimes, calcium.

Stenosis ⟿ A blockage in a coronary artery, caused by a plaque; classified as mild, moderate, or severe, or expressed as a percentage. An artery can become 70 percent blocked before symptoms of angina appear. Blockages of 20 to 50 percent are a sign of early disease, do not necessarily result in angina, and are usually treated with medication and diet.

Left main disease ⟿ Disease in the left (main) coronary artery, the most important blood vessel of the heart. If this vessel is severely diseased, bypass surgery is usually recommended, although angioplasty may be possible.

Occlusion ⟿ A total blockage (100 percent) of the vessel. Chronic occlusions (a blockage over 6 months old) can be very difficult to unblock by angioplasty. Even if successful, the re-narrowing rate after angioplasty is higher. Bypass surgery is often preferred in this situation.

Impaired left ventricular function ⟿ The pumping action of the main chamber of the heart (the left ventricle). This is often impaired after a heart attack and can strongly influence whether you have angioplasty or bypass surgery.

The Downside of Angiography 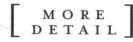 [**MORE DETAIL**]

The main benefit of coronary angiography is that it gives a clear picture of your heart disease and allows your physician to recommend treatment that is right for you. However, as with all medical procedures, there are risks and you should be aware of these before giving your consent for surgery (for more on patient consent, see page 38).

- Severe bleeding or bruising happens in about 1 in 100 people.

- The radio-opaque dye can occasionally lead to allergic reactions (about 1 in 1,000 people) or deterioration in the function of your kidneys (especially in people with pre-existing kidney disease).

- It is not common, but there may be infection, pain, or blockage of the blood vessel at the site of the puncture.

- Very occasionally the catheters can damage one of the heart's blood vessels, or, in about 2 in 1,000 people, cause a stroke.

- Angina can occur during the procedure, but this is un-common. If it does, inform the nurse and cardiologist immediately.

- One in 100 people suffer abnormal heartbeats during the procedure.

- As with all X-rays, there is exposure to radiation. One coronary angiogram is equivalent to approximately fifteen trans-Atlantic flights.

- Finally, some people suffer a heart attack or die during or after the procedure, but this is rare and happens in fewer than 1 in 1,000 people.

Chapter 3

is angioplasty right for you?

What Happens in this Chapter

- How your physician decides
  which treatment to recommend
- Your other options
- Pros and cons of angioplasty,
  bypass surgery, and medication alone

*If you have angina, you do not necessarily have to have
angioplasty. There are other options that can get the blood
flowing into your heart muscle again. Not all these treatments
will be suitable for your own situation, however, and your
medical team may strongly recommend one over another.
In general, the more disease in your blood vessels, the more
likely it is that you will be recommended for bypass surgery
rather than angioplasty or medication alone.*

The Treatment Decision

ONCE YOUR CORONARY ANGIOGRAM AND OTHER TESTS HAVE confirmed that you have angina, you and your physician will need to agree on the best treatment. Angina can be treated with either drug therapy, angioplasty, or coronary artery bypass surgery. Your physician will make a recommendation based on his or her past experience with patients whose medical situation is similar to yours, the number of factors in your life that may affect the health of your heart (for example, obesity), whether or not you have any other serious medical or surgical conditions, and his or her knowledge of the most recent scientific studies.

Your state of health may mean that the choice is obvious. For instance, you may have had a heart attack due to a blockage that can easily be cleared with angioplasty. More commonly, the decision is less clear-cut and you will be able to go with your own preference. If there is no particular medical reason to choose one treatment over another, the decision may depend on practical considerations, such as locally available hospital resources and how quickly you need to return to work.

This chapter summarizes the advantages and disadvantages of drug therapy, bypass surgery, and angioplasty, based on the most recently available scientific information. Our intention is to give you enough information to be able to make an informed decision about your treatment. If you prefer to leave the decision-making to your physician, that's fine, too.

"I saw others walking around after their angioplasty and thought, 'It can't be too bad if they're all OK.' Other patients in hospital said it wasn't too bad and it was helpful having someone to talk to. You realize it's a common procedure and lots of other people have it."

Bill Hogarth

How to Decide?

- Your own health situation may mean that one or more of the options in this chapter are not available to you. However, it's still worth knowing the advantages and disadvantages of your own treatment so that you are fully informed before you sign the consent form.

- If in doubt, a second opinion from another physician can sometimes help.

- As with all illnesses, your heart disease can change over time and you may need to revise your decision.

- You are entitled to change your mind if you feel that you have made the wrong choice.

- For more information on bypass surgery, see the book, *So You're Having Heart Bypass Surgery...What Happens Next?* (see page 145).

Drug Treatment

All patients with angina are treated with medication, whether they choose to have angioplasty or not. You may be on many drugs, some to relieve your angina, others to reduce the risks of a heart attack, and still others aimed at slowing the progression of your heart disease, including drugs to lower your cholesterol and blood pressure (for a detailed discussion of medications, see Chapter 12).

With the large number of potent and effective anti-angina drugs currently available, many patients with mild or moderate angina can be successfully treated by drug therapy alone. You may choose to simply manage your angina by continuing with, or adding to, your existing medication.

Obviously, the main advantage of treating your angina with medication alone is that you don't have to undergo the pain or inconvenience of a hospital procedure.

The main disadvantage of dealing with your angina by drug treatment alone is the sheer number of medications you may have to take. By contrast, after a successful angioplasty or bypass surgery you may be able to cut down on the number of drugs you take because you will no longer need to take medication for your angina symptoms.

The greater the number of drugs you take and the higher their doses, the more likely you are to suffer drug side effects. A list of the common side effects associated with heart medications is given in Chapter 12. It is impossible for your physician to predict whether you will suffer any side effects. Bear in mind, too, that it is impossible for him or her to give any guarantees about how well your angina will respond to medication, or which drug will be most effective. A period of trial and error is often needed before your physician can find the right combination of drugs—and doses—to suit you.

Despite these limitations, drug therapy may be the right long-term option for you if you are unhappy about the risks of a hospital procedure and if your angina is well controlled—that is, if your angina attacks are infrequent and you can lead a normal or near-normal life with few or no restrictions.

Remember, if your angina gets worse in the future, you can always change your mind and ask your physician to refer you for angioplasty or bypass surgery.

What Is Angioplasty?

Angioplasty involves unblocking your narrowed coronary arteries by inserting a small balloon into each artery and inflating the balloon at the site of the blockage. This presses the blockage to the sides of the artery and stretches (dilates) the artery slightly, allowing blood to flow freely once more. It involves making a small incision (cut) in either the arm or the groin to insert the balloon equipment all the way up to the heart. (For more on the angioplasty procedure, see Chapter 6.)

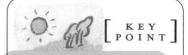

[KEY POINT]

If your angina is NOT well controlled by your medication, for example, if you experience angina when doing nothing to provoke an attack, or you suffer recurrent or prolonged episodes of angina, you should tell your doctor.

What is Bypass Surgery?

Coronary artery bypass surgery was first performed in 1968 and has since undergone many improvements. A heart surgeon creates a "bypass" around the blocked coronary artery by using a length of blood vessel taken from either the leg or chest. The resulting bypass is called a **coronary artery bypass graft** or **CABG** (pronounced "cabbage"). Thus, bypass surgery does not attempt to unblock the coronary arteries—it simply creates another route for the blood to reach the heart muscle. For more on bypass surgery, see the book, *So You're Having Heart Bypass Surgery...What Happens Next?* (details on page 145).

"I managed for years on just medication until my bypass, although I was never free from my angina."

Robert (Bobby) Frew

The Advantages of Angioplasty

Simpler Procedure

The main advantage of angioplasty over bypass surgery is that it is quicker and less traumatic. An angioplasty procedure takes around 1 to 2 hours to perform, depending on the number of blockages and how complicated they are—sometimes even less. You are awake the whole time, and only a small incision in either your groin or arm is involved. This means that you recover fairly quickly. Bypass operations can take 3 to 4 hours to perform, involve opening up your chest, and you may take weeks or months to recover. Not surprisingly, angioplasty is often the choice of people who have major responsibilities at home or work.

No General Anesthetic

Bypass surgery requires a general anesthetic. Angioplasty uses only a local anesthetic injection and a mild sedative that you take by mouth. This means that you avoid the risks of a general anesthetic and your recovery period is much shorter.

No Grafts

Bypass surgery involves grafting a vein or artery from elsewhere in the body onto the heart to bypass the blocked artery. The pieces of vein or artery used for the bypass are called **conduits**. These are usually taken from leg veins or from arteries behind the breastbone. By contrast, angioplasty does not need conduits, so there is less pain and discomfort, and, again, the whole procedure is much simpler. In addition, it is sometimes hard to find suitable conduits in people with medical conditions such as varicose veins or lung disease. Angioplasty does not have these limitations.

Less Chance of a Blood Transfusion

A blood transfusion is rarely needed for coronary angioplasty, but is more common if you undergo bypass surgery. Only in the unlikely situation that you have severe and life-threatening bleeding during angioplasty—for instance, as a result of all the blood-thinning medication you receive—will a blood transfusion be needed. Because such bleeding complications during angioplasty are so rare, blood is not routinely cross-matched (see Glossary) prior to your procedure, although a sample of your blood will be sent to the hospital laboratory to be held ready for testing in case an emergency arises.

Shorter Hospital Stay

After routine bypass surgery, patients generally stay in the hospital about 5 days. If all goes well, with an angioplasty, you will be out of the hospital the next day.

Less Risk (for some patients)

Up to 1 in 50 people having bypass surgery suffer a mild stroke. For angioplasty, the risk is about 1 in 200 (for more on risks, see pages 31 and 34).

Quicker Recovery

Angioplasty is less traumatic than a bypass operation, so the total recovery time (both in the hospital and at home) is shorter. Immediately after bypass surgery you will be transferred, still unconscious, to the intensive care unit. By contrast, after angioplasty, you will be fully conscious and will spend just a few hours in a special recovery area, then go home the next day.

Once home, the site of the incision will take a few days to fully heal, but you should return to normal very quickly. You may take weeks or months to return to normal following bypass surgery.

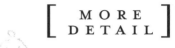

*Angioplasty **may** be a better option for you than bypass surgery if you have*

[**MORE DETAIL**]

- had a very recent heart attack
- varicose veins
- lung disease (e.g., asthma or bronchitis)
- any medical condition that means you shouldn't have a general anesthetic
- had a past stroke
- kidney disease
- diseased arteries elsewhere in the body (circulation problems)
- had one or more coronary bypass grafts already

The Downsides of Angioplasty

A Temporary Measure?

In general, angioplasty is very effective for treating symptoms of angina, but there is no evidence, at present, that it prevents heart attacks or will extend your life expectancy. Therefore, if you have an angioplasty you may still run the risk of your angina returning, or of suffering a heart attack in the future. No one is sure why this is, but it may have something to do with the fact that angioplasty does not remove the disease from all the blood vessel, which may cause problems in the future. By contrast, bypass surgery, which bypasses the entire diseased blood vessel, can prevent heart attacks *in some people*. These include people with severe disease of the left main artery, or disease of all three arteries *and* a weakened left ventricle, or diabetic people with disease in two or more blood vessels.

This consideration may swing you in favor of bypass surgery, especially if you are young or have a young family, but bear in mind that this apparent advantage is based on studies done before recent advances in angioplasty technology, such as **stents**—now a routine part of most angioplasties. Because of this, it is difficult to truly compare current angioplasty procedures and bypass surgery. They may turn out to be equally effective. Studies are currently underway to compare bypass surgery with stents in the long term.

> "I loved the whole experience. I said, 'Can I watch the procedure?' and they said, 'Yes.' What I didn't enjoy was my recovery."
>
> **Arni Cohn**

Risks of the Procedure

Angioplasty, like all medical procedures, carries a risk of complications—unwanted medical events that happen during or after the procedure. Some people are more at risk of complications than others and not all of the risks described below will apply to you. If you want some indication of your personal risks, talk to your physician.

The main risks of angioplasty and bypass surgery are shown in the More Detail box on page 34. Doctors divide risks into "early" complications (within hours or days) and "late" (long-term) complications.

The most frequent **early complication** is some bleeding or bruising at the incision site. Less common early complications are an aneurysm, where blood leaks out of the blood vessel at the site of the incision, or collapse of the coronary artery, due to the balloon tearing the artery wall during angioplasty. Sudden blockages in one or more coronary arteries can also occur during the procedure. This can lead to a small heart attack in 2 to 5 out of every 100 patients.

The most potentially serious early complication of angioplasty is a condition called **stent thrombosis**, where a blood clot forms on the metal stent, causing a blockage in the coronary artery and, thus, a heart attack. In the past, this complication occurred in up to 5 percent of patients after stent insertion. Nowadays, thanks to potent

*You **may** benefit more from bypass surgery than angioplasty if you have:*

[**MORE DETAIL**]

- a coronary artery that has been completely blocked for several weeks or months
- damaged heart valves or other condition that requires heart surgery
- coronary arteries narrowed in more than one place
- blockages in all three coronary arteries AND a weakened left ventricle
- diabetes AND more than one blocked artery

drugs that prevent blood clotting (see page 52), and improved techniques of stent implantation, stent thrombosis occurs in less than 1 percent of people. Because of the potential for stent thrombosis, anti-platelet drugs must be continued for a minimum of 1 month after angioplasty to allow the blood vessel to cover the stent with the normal blood vessel lining.

In the long term, the most serious potential **late complication** of angioplasty is a condition called **re-stenosis**, where the coronary artery blocks up again several weeks or months later. This usually causes angina to return. This occurs in 20 to 30 percent of patients following balloon angioplasty alone, and 10 to 20 percent of patients who have had a stent inserted.

For more on weighing up the risks of angioplasty, see page 38, Consent.

What Happens Next?

There are many factors to consider when trying to decide between medication alone and a hospital procedure, or between bypass surgery and angioplasty. If you are having trouble deciding, it may be worth seeking a second opinion from another physician. Don't feel embarrassed to do this because, at the end of the day you will be the one undergoing angioplasty or bypass surgery, not your doctor.

It is worth remembering, too, that angioplasty and bypass surgery can relieve your angina, but neither procedure actually cures your heart disease. Even if you have angioplasty or bypass surgery, you still need to make changes that will improve the health of your heart, otherwise your heart disease will continue to get worse. Take your medication correctly and don't forget to make lifestyle changes (see Chapter 10). Heart disease is a wake-up call: it's time to choose a different road.

> "The doctor was always in a hurry; I wish he could have spent more time with me. I'd rather hear about the risks, then make up my own mind."
>
> **Robert (Bobby) Frew**

Major Risks of Coronary (Heart) Bypass Surgery

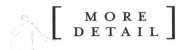

[**MORE DETAIL**]

- Death (less than 1 percent)
- Heart attack (2 to 6 percent)
- Stroke (1 to 2 percent)

Major Risks of Angioplasty

- Death (less than 0.1 percent)
- Heart attack (2 to 5 percent)
- Stroke (0.5 percent)
- Bleeding or bruising serious enough to need a blood transfusion or surgical repair (less than 0.5 percent)
- Sudden blockage of coronary artery, resulting in emergency bypass surgery (less than 1 percent)

Chapter 4

getting ready for your angioplasty

What Happens in this Chapter

- Tests you'll need before your angioplasty
- Consent
- Questions you may want to ask

Preparing for your angioplasty not only involves hospital tests and procedures, but also things that you can do for yourself. This is a good time to read up on your procedure so that you can prepare any questions you may wish to ask before you sign the consent form. You can also use the time to make practical arrangements for your hospital visit.

Planning for Angioplasty

ONCE YOU HAVE AGREED TO HAVE AN ANGIOPLASTY, THE LENGTH of time you will have to wait depends on three factors:

1) the severity of your symptoms

2) how badly your coronary arteries are narrowed

3) the number of other patients on your physician's waiting list

If the circumstances are right, you may be able to have angioplasty the same day as your angiogram (see "ad-hoc angioplasty," page 20).

If you have a long time to wait, you may wish to start some of the self-help techniques in Chapter 10.

Pre-Angioplasty Tests

A small number of blood tests and an ECG (see Glossary) are usually performed before your angioplasty. These blood tests include checking to see how your kidneys are working and whether you are anemic. The good news is that, if you have already had several blood tests before your angiogram, only one extra test is required for an angioplasty. This involves taking a sample of blood to be held in reserve in case you need a blood transfusion during or following your angioplasty. This blood sample will be used to match donor blood to you, in the unlikely event of an emergency.

"Before the angioplasty they offered me counseling to help me cope. I refused it—it's normal to be having these problems at age 71."

Mrs. C.V.

Pre-Angioplasty Arrangements

The amount of time you will need off work for your angioplasty depends partly on how physically demanding your occupation is. If it involves heavy or strenuous exercise, you will need at least 7 days off, particularly if you are having your angioplasty via your groin. This reduces the chance of further bleeding or bruising at the incision site when you do return to work. If your job is fairly sedentary, it may be safe for you to return to work as early as the following day, if you wish. You can also get back to work faster if you are having your angioplasty via your wrist. Bear in mind, too, that you will not be able to drive for a few days after your angioplasty, so this may affect how early you can return to work.

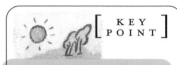

[KEY POINT]

You may not be able to get insurance to fly until at least 3 months after your angioplasty. Bear this in mind when booking your angioplasty, if you are given a choice of dates.

Some patients like to tidy up their paperwork at home before coming into the hospital for their angioplasty. Sorting out financial loose ends and updating your will are some suggestions. These kinds of preparations give many people a sense of comfort. While this may or may not be right for you, it is worth considering.

Although this is not specifically related to angioplasty, some patients also like to draw up a "living will." A living will clearly informs your family and your physician about exactly what you would like, and, probably more importantly, would *not* like, in case you fall into a coma. Again, you may not wish to pursue this: it is just something to think about.

"I wasn't at all worried because my husband had already had angioplasty twice. I knew about the procedure and I also had one hundred percent faith in my doctor."

Mrs. C.V.

Consent

Before you have your angioplasty, you will need to give your written consent. This is one of the most important steps of your angioplasty procedure.

What Exactly Is "Consent"?

You make decisions to take risks every day of your life. Some kind of risk is involved when you cross a road, place a bet on a horse, drive your car, or board an airplane. However, when you go into the hospital to have an operation, the risk you take feels different because you are allowing somebody else, usually a doctor, to make decisions for you. Nonetheless, it is a risk just like every other part of life. Although the physician will be acting in your best interest, it is still important that you understand exactly what you are giving your permission for, or consent to. You are therefore entitled to know what is going to happen to you, why the procedure is needed, and what the risks are. If you agree to having angioplasty, you have given your consent.

You may be asked for your consent for your angioplasty operation on the day of the procedure or in a pre-admission clinic. Either way, it is an important part of your angioplasty experience that can sometimes cause further anxiety and lead to misunderstanding. It is crucial that you read the consent form and understand what it is you are signing. Do not feel pressured to sign the consent form immediately. Take at least a few moments to read through it and, if there is enough time you can always take the form home and bring it back on the day of your procedure. Most consent forms will have paragraphs in them saying that the physician may carry out additional procedures should the need arise (for example, in an emergency situation, or if your heart disease has worsened since your

> "The night before they give you something to help you sleep a bit, but I wasn't overly concerned or nervous. They showed me a diagram and there were videos about what they were going to do."
>
> **Bill Hogarth**

angiogram). Ask your physician or the
nurse, if you can, what additional
procedures may be carried out and what
the possible outcomes of these procedures
might be. If you are worried about any
part of the procedure, or you feel you

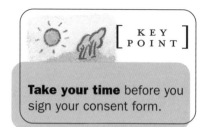

[**KEY POINT**]

Take your time before you
sign your consent form.

have not received a clear answer on anything, now is the time to say so.
Once you have signed the consent form, it will be assumed that you
understand everything about your procedure and the risks involved.

Risks of Angioplasty

Because angioplasty involves an operation on an organ as complex as
your heart, there are a number of potential complications—unwanted
medical events—that may occur during or after the procedure (see
pages 31 and 34).

Bear in mind that risks are only estimates, and you are unlikely to
have any of these complications. Your physician will certainly be doing

Consent 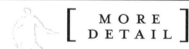 [**MORE DETAIL**]

There are three types of consent:

Implied consent ⟿ usually reserved for minor procedures, such
as blood tests or having a tongue depressor put into your mouth.
In these cases, you non-verbally comply by sticking your arm out or
opening your mouth.

Verbal consent ⟿ can be used in an emergency situation, when
there is no time to obtain a signature on a consent form.

Written consent ⟿ needed before medical procedures that
require an anesthetic because you will be given drugs that make
you drowsy or put you to sleep. Since you will not be able to give
your consent to your physician during your procedure, written consent—a legally binding document—is needed before the operation.

Questions Commonly Asked by Patients About to Undergo Angioplasty

1. Am I at greater risk of having a stroke or a heart attack during the procedure?
2. Do you intend to use a stent and, if so, how many?
3. How many blood vessels are you going to angioplasty?
4. Will I be able to reduce my medication afterwards?
5. Will you use any other devices during the angioplasty?
6. What are the chances of my stent blocking in the future?
7. Will I feel any pain during the procedure?

You may also like to use the Patient Diary at the back of the book to write your own questions.

his or her best to prevent them. To estimate your own particular risk, your physician takes into account the exact state of your heart's arteries (from your coronary angiogram), the severity of your blockage(s), and the size of the diseased coronary artery. The risks associated with your angioplasty can also be affected by the strength (or weakness) of your heart's muscle and any other medical conditions (for example, asthma or diabetes) that you may have. For a full description of the factors that can reduce or increase the risks of angioplasty, see Chapter 3.

Asking Questions

Feel free to ask any questions you like before signing your consent form. Reading up on angioplasty beforehand is helpful because you will understand more of what you are being told and be able to come up with questions more easily (see also Self Help box).

What Happens Next?

Once you have signed the consent form the next step is the angioplasty procedure itself.

Chapter 5

the day of your angioplasty

What Happens in this Chapter

- Making a hospital checklist
- Arrival at the hospital
- Tips for friends and family
- Medications you may be given
- Transfer to the cath lab

*Your big day finally arrives. It is normal for you to feel anxious on the day of your angioplasty, but good preparation helps. When you get to the hospital you will be assigned a bed and a nurse to look after you. There will be some routine tests and you will be given blood-thinning medication and a sedative. You will then be taken to the **cardiac catheterization laboratory (cath lab)** where your angioplasty will be carried out.*

Planning Your Day

THE MAJORITY OF PATIENTS WHO UNDERGO ANGIOPLASTY ARE
admitted the same morning as their procedure and discharged the
following day. Be sure to pack everything you will need to stay in the
hospital overnight, including a full list of your medications (you can
use the diary at the back of this book to write down your medicines).
Remember to make arrangements to be taken home from the hospital because you will be advised not to drive home yourself.

[S E L F - H E L P]

Hospital Checklist

This checklist may be useful before you leave for the
hospital:

✔

- Take ALL your medication with a sip of water. ◯
  Blood-thinning medication such as
  warfarin (Coumadin) should have
  been stopped 3 to 5 days before
  your procedure, unless you were
  specifically told to continue by your
  physician.
- Shave your groin. ◯
- Pack a full list of your medications. ◯
- Do not eat or drink anything, unless ◯
  specifically told that you can.
- Pack some reading material with you, but ◯
  forget about taking any work or business
  material. Sedative medication during your
  procedure will make you drowsy afterwards
  and unable to concentrate on work.

Hospital Arrival

When you arrive at the hospital you will be assigned a bed and a nurse to look after you. After you have changed into a hospital gown, an intravenous line will be inserted into one of your arms. This will be used to give you fluids and to administer drugs during and after the procedure. You will not be allowed to drink until after your procedure. You will then be examined by a physician, your consent for the operation will be obtained (see page 38), and routine blood tests and an ECG will be performed. You may have already gone through some of these steps on previous hospital visits.

While you are waiting for your angioplasty, there will be a nurse assigned to look after you (and a number of other patients). Now is the time to tell the nurse about any anxieties or unanswered questions you have.

"They took me to the hospital by ambulance the day before and, after the blood work, etc., first thing in the morning I had my angioplasty. It took about 45 minutes to 1 hour and you're awake the whole time... it's not long."

Bill Hogarth

Medication Before Your Procedure

Blood Thinners

Blood clotting is a natural process where **platelets** (tiny cell fragments in the blood) and special blood proteins bind together to form a clot. It is a lifesaver at the right time and in the right place (for instance, after an injury), but is dangerous when it happens inside blood vessels. In this case, the blood clot could block the vessel and cut off blood flow, causing a heart attack. Blood clots are more likely to form when the blood flow meets an obstruction or makes contact with an

Self-Help on the Day

- Try to deal with any problems or questions you may have *before* you go into the cath lab for your angioplasty. The cath lab team is concentrating on making your procedure a success and may be too preoccupied to answer questions.

- Do not be afraid to ask for additional sedation. Proper sedation in the cardiac catheterization laboratory can make the procedure easier for both you and your physician.

- For more information on getting settled in the cath lab, see Chapter 2.

"The patient's attitude is 100 percent responsible for the care they get... 100 percent. If you're a happy, smiling, cooperative patient, the nurse will come when you want them to. If there's any other attitude, unfortunately, you will end up waiting. Maybe not too long, but you will end up waiting. It's human nature."

Arni Cohn

injury on the artery wall. Both these situations are common during angioplasty, so you will need **blood-thinning medication** to ensure that all is well during the procedure.

To successfully prevent blood clotting—either in your blood vessels or on the angioplasty equipment—the activity of both the platelets and the blood-clotting proteins must be blocked.

You may already be taking ASA (Aspirin), a very common and inexpensive blood-thinner used by patients with coronary heart disease. ASA works by blocking the activity of platelets.

For this reason, it is called an **anti-platelet drug**. Although ASA is effective in preventing most blood-clotting problems that happen after balloon angioplasty, it is less effective when a stent is used. Approximately 3 to 5 percent of stents (mesh-like supports placed inside coronary arteries) will block suddenly in the first week after angioplasty due to the formation of a blood clot inside the stent. To reduce the chances of this happening, additional anti-platelet drugs will be given to you when you have an angioplasty with a stent, such as ticlopidine (Ticlid) and clopidogrel (Plavix).

"I got to the hospital early in the morning and my turn came at 10 am. I was back in my room an hour later."

Mrs. C.V.

Ticlopidine or clopidogrel are usually given to you as tablets before your procedure and taken for a short period (usually 4 weeks) afterward. Both drugs work by further reducing the "stickiness" of platelets. Although ticlopidine and clopidogrel work in the same way, there are important differences between them when it comes to side effects. Ticlopidine can occasionally result in a reduction in the number of white cells in your blood due to its direct effect on the bone marrow. This will make you prone to infections. Fortunately, this is uncommon because ticlopidine is prescribed for only a short duration (usually 2 to 4 weeks) and routine blood counts by your family doctor will pick up any problems fairly quickly. Clopidogrel requires no such precautions.

Sedatives

Most patients feel a little anxious before their angioplasty and find that mild oral sedatives, given to them beforehand, are helpful. The type and dose of sedative medication will vary from hospital to hospital. If you feel that you are still anxious when you reach the cath lab and you need something stronger, a rapidly acting intravenous sedative drug can be given to you. Your sedative medication will make you drowsy, but you will still be conscious.

Transfer to the Cardiac Catheterization Laboratory (Cath lab)

Unless you are the first case of the day, the exact time of your procedure can only be estimated. While your nursing staff and doctors will do their best to give you some idea of when your procedure will take place, this will be affected by how long other patients' angioplasties take (which can be difficult to estimate) and whether there are any unexpected emergencies.

For more about arrival at the cath lab, and getting comfortable, see Chapter 2.

Friends and Family

Depending on individual hospital policy, your friends and family members may be allowed to stay with you before your angioplasty. This often helps to calm anxiety and will give you support when you're asking questions during the process of giving your consent.

Family and friends will not be allowed to stay with you after your transfer to the cath lab. During your angioplasty, there is often a special waiting area for friends and family. If they do not want to remain in the waiting area, suggest to them that they leave details of how they can be contacted with the nursing staff, in the unlikely event that a member of your medical team wishes to speak with them during your angioplasty. Because the time required for an angioplasty can vary greatly, from 30 minutes to 3 hours, no guarantee can be given about when you will be transferred back to the ward.

What Happens Next?

Once you are in the cath lab, your angioplasty can begin.

Chapter 6

the angioplasty procedure

What Happens in this Chapter

- A step-by-step guide to your coronary angioplasty procedure
- Angiography during the procedure
- Use of blood-thinning drugs
- Insertion of the guide wire
- Balloon angioplasty
- Insertion of stents
- Closing the incision

Coronary angioplasty, a procedure used to treat angina and heart attacks, was first performed in the late 1970s. It involves widening blocked coronary arteries by inflating a small balloon within the blocked region of the artery. Many sophisticated technologies have been added to this basic procedure over the years, including metal stents to keep the artery open, drills and cutters to remove blockages, and sophisticated blood-thinning drugs to improve patient safety. As a result of these improvements, angioplasty is now performed safely and effectively in the vast majority of patients, who can avoid bypass surgery and benefit from a quick recovery.

What is Coronary Angioplasty?

ANGIOPLASTY IS A TECHNIQUE USED TO WIDEN ANY ARTERY THAT has become blocked by fatty deposits in the artery walls. Coronary angioplasty is angioplasty of the coronary arteries—the crucial arteries that supply blood to the heart muscle. The procedure involves inserting a tube called a **guide catheter** into a major artery in the groin or wrist, then up to the heart and into the affected artery (see Figure 5). A thin wire (**guide wire**) is then passed down the guide catheter and across the blockage itself. A balloon is passed along the wire and inflated at the point of the obstruction. This not only crushes the blockage against the sides of the artery, but also stretches the artery slightly, to widen it (see Figure 7). Often, a small metal tube called a **stent** is permanently placed in the artery to help keep the artery open (see Figure 9).

The technical term for coronary angioplasty is **percutaneous transluminal coronary angioplasty**, or **PTCA**, because the guide wire and the balloon pass through a small incision in the skin ("percutaneous") and into the interior, or **lumen**, of the artery ("transluminal").

Getting Ready

If you have already had a coronary angiogram, the **cardiac catheterization laboratory**, or **cath lab**, and the first few steps of your angioplasty procedure will be familiar to you (see Chapter 2). You will make yourself comfortable on the table in the cath lab and have ECG leads attached to your chest. You will then receive a small local-anesthetic injection into your skin and a short plastic tube called a **sheath** will be inserted into a small incision in your groin or, if you are having angioplasty via your arm, in your wrist.

Your Angioplasty Procedure

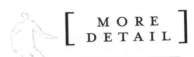

The following are the basic steps of your coronary angioplasty. If you have already had an angiogram, steps 1 to 4 will be familiar.

1. A local anesthetic injection is given into the skin above a blood vessel in your groin or arm.

2. A small incision is made through the skin, following which a needle is inserted into the blood vessel.

3. A sheath (small plastic tube) is placed into the blood vessel, through which the guide catheter is inserted.

4. The guide catheter is passed all the way to the coronary arteries of the heart.

5. A repeat coronary angiography is done (see Chapter 2).

6. Blood-thinning medication is administered.

7. A guide wire is passed through the guiding catheter and across the blocked region of the coronary artery ("wiring the vessel").

8. The angioplasty balloon travels along the wire into the narrowed blood vessel.

9. The balloon is inflated and deflated to widen the artery.

10. The stent implantation is performed (if required).

11. Other procedures are performed (if required).

12. The incision is closed.

Guiding Catheter

After the sheath is in place, a narrow tube called a guiding catheter will be inserted through the sheath and into your leg or arm artery, all the way to your heart (see Figure 5). As the name implies, all the equipment for your angioplasty will pass through this guiding catheter, just as a subway train runs through a tunnel (see Figure 6). Once the guiding catheter is in place, the procedure can begin.

Figure 5. Cardiac Catheterization

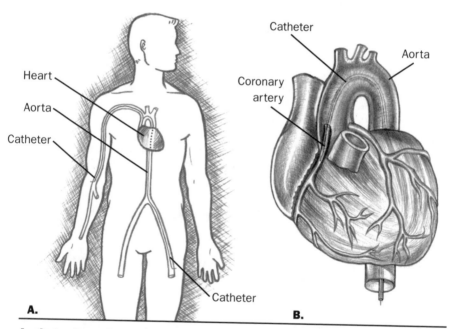

A.   **B.**

Angiography and angioplasty use this technique, in which a tube called a catheter is inserted into the heart's blood vessels via an artery in the arm or the groin (A). The catheter is then used to inject radio-opaque dye and insert angioplasty equipment into the coronary arteries (B).

The Angioplasty Equipment

Although you may not be aware of it during the procedure, angioplasty uses equipment that is slightly different from that used during your coronary angiogram. First, the diameter of the catheters may be larger since some specialized and bulky angioplasty equipment requires extra-large catheters. Second, the guiding catheters are stiffer to provide extra support to the angioplasty equipment. As a result, it may take longer to insert the tip of the angioplasty guiding catheter into your narrowed blood vessel.

Repeat Coronary Angiography

Your angioplasty procedure will start with your doctor taking a few more angiogram pictures of your narrowed blood vessel or vessels. He or she does this to confirm that there have been no major changes since your previous coronary angiogram. The new pictures will also help him or her select the correct size and length of balloons and stents to be used during your procedure.

Nitroglycerin, which you currently use to treat your angina attacks, may be injected directly down your narrowed coronary artery to help it relax before the angiogram pictures are taken.

Angiography will also be used throughout your procedure to guide your physician and to assess the results of the balloon inflation or stent insertion.

> "They give you Ativan to relax you. There's a burning sensation in the groin when they cut, but it's not really painful. Once in a while he'd move it, and it would feel tender at the entry site, but there's no pain in the chest."
>
> **Bill Hogarth**

Blood-Thinning Medication During Your Angioplasty

For more on blood thinners, see page 43.

Heparin

Heparin blocks the action of the blood-clotting proteins. It is given intravenously (into your vein) during your angioplasty and, in combination with your oral blood-thinning medication, such as ASA, clopidogrel, or ticlopidine (pages 43–45), will significantly reduce your blood's ability to clot.

Special Blood Thinners

Recently, a new type of anti-platelet drug has been found to be useful in patients undergoing angioplasty. These drugs are known by

Glycoprotein IIB/IIIA Inhibitors
e.g., abciximab (ReoPro), eptifibatide
(Integrillin), tirofiban (Aggrastat)

[**MORE DETAIL**]

These new, powerful anti-platelet drugs have been shown to be very effective in reducing the risk of a heart attack in patients undergoing angioplasty and reducing angina in severely ill patients. However, their use varies greatly between hospitals, due primarily to their high cost. They are often used only for patients undergoing "high-risk" or difficult angioplasties. These may include narrowings with blood clots or patients who have had a recent heart attack, heart failure, or diabetes, or patients who are elderly.

The main side effects that can occur with the use of these drugs are, as you would suspect, bleeding and bruising. Infrequent, but potentially serious, side effects include allergic reactions and, occasionally, a dramatic fall in the blood-platelet count. The use of such drugs, therefore, requires additional precautions, including extra blood tests during your hospital stay.

the long and complicated name of **glycoprotein IIb/IIIa** (or **2B-3A) inhibitors**. They act by blocking the clotting effects of platelets, but they are many times more powerful than oral blood thinners. These drugs are only available for intravenous injection and are used during, and for a short time after, angioplasty in some hospitals (see More Detail box).

To make sure that your blood is not over-thinned, a blood sample will be taken during your angioplasty for an **Activated Clotting Time (ACT)** test. The overall goal is to prevent blood clots, while, at the same time, making sure you do not suffer from bleeding complications. A balance is achieved in most cases, but bleeding or clotting complications do occur occasionally.

Insertion of the Guide Wire

The first important step during your angioplasty is "wiring the vessel." A long wire called a guide wire helps direct equipment such as balloons and stents into your narrowed blood vessel and through the actual narrowing (see Figure 6). The guide wire is first inserted into the guiding catheter and then, using the X-ray camera, its tip is carefully navigated down your blood vessel. You may see the guide wire moving down your blood vessel on the X-ray screen. Angioplasty guide wires are very small in diameter—only 36/1000 of a centimeter wide.

"I think the fact that you can see what's happening on the television tends to keep your mind off things because you're watching what's going on, rather than just lying there and letting them do their thing.... And of course they have a bit of music going and the nurses are talking to you."

Bill Hogarth

The insertion of a guide wire into a narrowed blood vessel rarely causes any problems, although it can sometimes cause angina symptoms. Occasionally, it is impossible for the physician to pass a guide wire through the narrowed region of a blood vessel. If this happens, it means, unfortunately, that your angioplasty cannot go ahead because *all* angioplasty equipment needs a correctly positioned guide wire. This is more common if your blood vessel is totally blocked, rather than just narrowed, particularly if the complete blockage is more than a few months old.

Figure 6. Keeping Angioplasty on Track

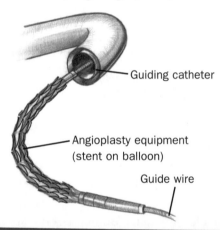

Guiding catheter

Angioplasty equipment
(stent on balloon)

Guide wire

Just as a train runs on tracks through a subway tunnel, the angioplasty equipment travels to your heart on a guide wire through a guiding tube or catheter. The guide wire keeps the equipment on track as it moves into position at the site of blockage.

Balloon Angioplasty

Once the guide wire is passed across the blockage, the next step is usually the use of an angioplasty balloon. Your physician will insert the balloon along the guide wire and into your narrowed blood vessel. Angioplasty balloons were invented by a Swiss physician, Dr. Andreas Gruntzig, in the late 1970s. They are now available in a huge range of diameters and lengths, and your doctor will select one that exactly fits your blood vessel. These tough, plastic balloons can withstand pressure of up to 20 atmospheres and are designed to inflate to precisely the right diameter.

Once the balloon is inserted along the guide wire and into the narrowed area of your blood vessel, it will be inflated and deflated, using a hand-held pump (see Figures 7 and 8). The balloon is inflated with fluid visible on the X-ray screen (not air), so the physician can watch it as it expands and contracts.

Be forewarned: *angina symptoms at this stage are very common* because the inflated balloon temporarily blocks the flow of blood down the artery. Because the balloon is often inflated and deflated several times, you may feel angina pain coming and going. Your doctor should warn you each time you are likely to experience angina during your procedure.

Figure 7. Balloon Angioplasty

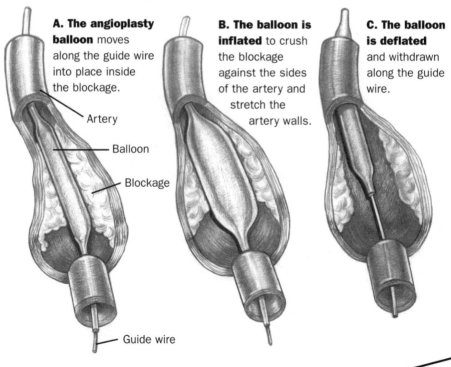

A. The angioplasty balloon moves along the guide wire into place inside the blockage.

Artery

Balloon

Blockage

Guide wire

B. The balloon is inflated to crush the blockage against the sides of the artery and stretch the artery walls.

C. The balloon is deflated and withdrawn along the guide wire.

Figure 8. Angioplasty Balloons

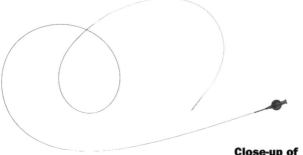

Angioplasty balloon and catheter

Close-up of angioplasty balloon before inflation

Inflated angioplasty balloon

Self-Help During Angioplasty

Also see the self-help advice for angiography, page 12.

If you experience any symptoms AT ANY STAGE of your angioplasty procedure, inform your physician or nurse right away. You may experience a headache after the nitroglycerin is injected into the blood vessels. Do not be alarmed, you will feel better as time passes.

Stents

Stents are metal coils or tubes that are used to try to improve the results of your angioplasty procedure. Studies show that angina returns in only 15 percent of Canadian patients who have stents inserted—up to half the rate for balloon angioplasty alone. Stents have also dramatically reduced the number of patients who need emergency bypass surgery after angioplasty. Although stenting does not provide perfect results, it is a definite improvement over balloon angioplasty alone. Whether you receive one or more stents depends on the size of your narrowed blood vessel and how long the narrowing is.

Early stents were relatively bulky and inflexible, so angioplasty physicians had to pre-stretch the narrowing with a balloon before inserting the stent. Modern stents can usually be inserted into a narrowed blood vessel without prior balloon angioplasty. This technique is called **direct stenting**.

A stent is usually delivered to the site of the blockage on an angioplasty balloon. As the balloon inflates, the stent enlarges and presses up against the sides of the blood vessel. Once the balloon is deflated and removed from the blood vessel, the stent is left behind to hold the walls of the blood vessel fully open (see Figures 9 and 10). Your physician may insert larger angioplasty balloons after your stent has been inserted to ensure full expansion of the stent—and a better long-term result. A small number of stents are self-expanding and do not require a balloon for insertion (although a balloon may be used to ensure that they are fully expanded) (see Figure 11).

Any symptoms that you may experience as a stent is put in place are similar to those of normal balloon angioplasty. You will not feel the stent being expanded or be aware of it afterwards. In the following months, the artery wall will gradually grow over the stent and cover it completely.

Although many different types of stents are available, there are few differences among them with respect to long-term results. On the whole, the long-term results of your angioplasty and stent will depend mainly on the size of your blood vessel and the length of the narrowed region. The type of stent that you will receive will depend upon which stent is available in your hospital and which stent your physician feels is most suitable for your blood vessel.

One of the downsides of stents is that they can suddenly block with a blood clot 3 to 5 days after angioplasty—a condition called **stent thrombosis** (see page 31). Stents can also be difficult to unblock if they become narrowed in the future.

Figure 9. Stent Insertion

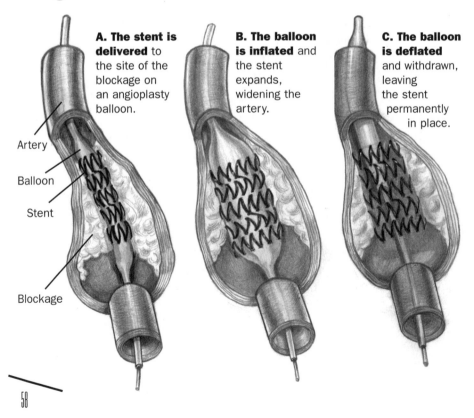

A. The stent is delivered to the site of the blockage on an angioplasty balloon.

B. The balloon is inflated and the stent expands, widening the artery.

C. The balloon is deflated and withdrawn, leaving the stent permanently in place.

Artery

Balloon

Stent

Blockage

Figure 10. Stents

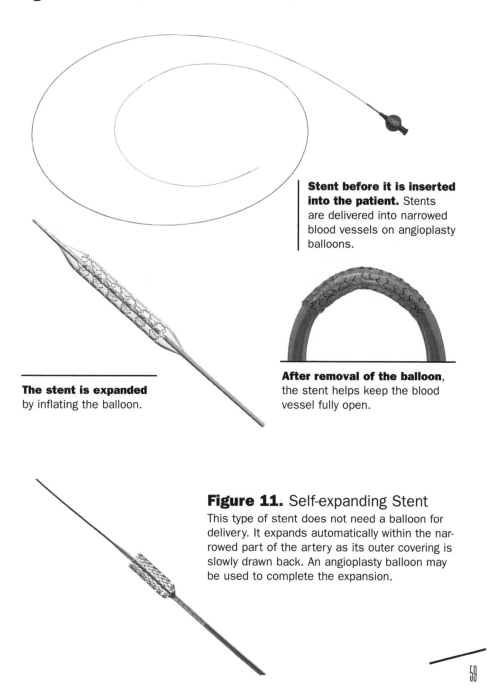

Stent before it is inserted into the patient. Stents are delivered into narrowed blood vessels on angioplasty balloons.

The stent is expanded by inflating the balloon.

After removal of the balloon, the stent helps keep the blood vessel fully open.

Figure 11. Self-expanding Stent

This type of stent does not need a balloon for delivery. It expands automatically within the narrowed part of the artery as its outer covering is slowly drawn back. An angioplasty balloon may be used to complete the expansion.

Other Angioplasty Techniques

Apart from balloons and stents, there is an increasing number of sophisticated angioplasty tools and techniques that your physician can use to help you. These are covered in Chapter 7, along with their advantages and disadvantages.

Closing the Incision

After your coronary angiogram, the sheath in your groin was probably removed immediately and the blood vessel left to form a clot before you were allowed out of bed. Unfortunately, this will not happen after your angioplasty. Because of all the blood-thinning medication you were given for your angioplasty, you are at a higher risk of bleeding immediately after your angioplasty than after your angiogram. What happens next will depend on whether your wrist or groin was used and whether your physician uses a closure device.

"During the procedure they gave me a picture of before and after, of what the artery looked like before and what they did."

Mrs. C.V.

Conventional Approach—Late Sheath Removal

If you have had angioplasty via your groin, the standard approach is to leave the sheath in place for 4 to 6 hours after your angioplasty, during which time you will be lying flat on your back in the recovery area (see page 71). This allows time for some of your blood-thinning medication to wear off.

Closure Devices—Immediate Sheath Removal

One of the alternatives to late sheath removal is the use of closure devices, which can halve the time you need to spend in bed. There are a number of different designs, but they all work basically the same way—by either plugging or tying shut the hole in your leg artery. Closure devices need to be put on in a sterile environment, so they are applied in the cath lab at the end of your angioplasty procedure. This usually adds only a few minutes to the end of your procedure. Closure devices allow you to move around a few hours after your angioplasty and, potentially, allow safe, early discharge from the hospital. Complications are uncommon with closure devices, but they do happen occasionally. These include damage to the artery or failure to prevent bleeding (in which case manual pressure may be used).

"They explained about pressure and the fact they had cut into a major artery and they had to seal the wound. The clamp looked like a huge vice, with one part underneath the mattress for stability. I was stuck in this big thing and thinking, 'I wonder who thought of this?'"

Arni Cohn

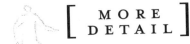

Angioplasty Via Your Wrist   [MORE DETAIL]

The technique of carrying out angioplasties via the wrist instead of the groin is growing in popularity, although it is still not used by all physicians and is not an option for some patients. Many physicians are not trained for the technique, and it is technically more difficult because the artery used (the radial artery) is much smaller than the one in the groin. With practice, physicians can perform most angioplasties equally well via the groin or the wrist.

To see whether you are able to have your angioplasty performed this way, the hospital will need to perform a simple circulation test called the **Allen's test** (see Glossary). This reveals whether you have one or two open blood vessels in your wrist. You will need two open blood vessels for wrist angioplasty.

The major advantage of wrist angioplasty for the patient is that he or she can sit up immediately after the procedure and will avoid a long period of bed rest—the most uncomfortable feature of angioplasty of the groin. The downside for the patient is that the insertion of the sheath can be painful due to the small size of the arteries.

Angioplasty Via the Wrist

If you had angioplasty via your wrist (see More Detail Box), the sheath is immediately removed by your physician when your angioplasty is over. Local pressure is then applied using either a compressive bandage or a wristband, and no closure devices are used.

Angioplasty Via the Elbow

This approach involves the blood vessel in your elbow (the **brachial artery**). It is gradually falling out of favor, although it may be useful in certain patients. The incision is closed by application of pressure or a suture.

At the End of Your Angioplasty

At the end of your angioplasty procedure, you should expect to be free of pain. If this is not the case, tell your physician. Very occasionally, an angioplasty patient may experience chest pain for a few hours after the procedure—for instance, due to blockage of a small side branch of your vessel caused by the balloon or stent. It is not always possible to keep all small side branches open when performing angioplasty. If this type of blockage occurs, it should be visible on your final angiogram pictures and your physician may prescribe pain-relieving medication. The pain should subside after a few hours. Very occasionally, this situation can result in a small heart attack. If this happens, it will be confirmed by blood tests taken the day after your angioplasty.

What Happens Next?

After your angioplasty is completed, you will be transferred to a special ward or recovery area. Here, you will learn how to care for your wound and how to take care of yourself while you are healing.

the angioplasty toolkit

What Happens in this Chapter

- A more detailed look at the tools your physician
  may use in the angioplasty procedure
- The low-down on atherectomy, thrombectomy, lasers
- Ancillary techniques your physician may use to help you

*There are a number of ways to improve the blood flow
down your narrowed or blocked arteries. Some are better
than others in terms of their short- and long-term results
and some are more suitable for certain kinds of narrowings than others. While you will not be able to choose the
tools that your physician selects, knowing something
about the angioplasty toolkit may help you feel more in
control of your procedure.*

Opening up the Toolkit

IN CHAPTER 6 WE LOOKED AT THE BASIC STEPS OF YOUR
angioplasty. You may feel that this is all you need (or want) to know
about your procedure. However, if you want more detail on the
sophisticated tools and techniques that your physician may use, this is
the chapter for you. You should come away with enough information
to understand what your doctor is telling you about techniques that
he or she will use during your procedure—and what questions to ask.

Atherectomy Devices

Neither balloon angioplasty nor stent insertion removes any of the
brittle, fatty blockage (**atherosclerotic plaque**) from the walls of
narrowed blood vessels. For this, cutting devices called **atherectomy
devices** are needed. Removing some of the plaque before balloon
angioplasty or stent insertion can make it easier for the physician to
inflate the balloon or open the stent completely.

A disadvantage of atherectomy devices in general is that they need
large guiding catheters that may be more uncomfortable for the
patient. There is also a slightly increased risk of complications, such
as heart attack, in part because atherectomy is traditionally used to
treat complex blockages.

Directional atherectomy devices incorporate a cutting blade and
balloon into the end of a catheter. They may prove to be particularly
useful in patients with a severe blockage on just one side of the
blood vessel wall or whose stents have become blocked. The latest
devices, such as the one in Figure 12, may be particularly helpful for
patients with a lot of calcium in their artery walls.

Rotational atherectomy devices are drill-like devices for remov-

Figure 12.
Directional
Atherectomy
Device
This combined balloon and cutter, called the FLEXI-CUT™ Directional Debulking System, slices plaque off the blood vessel wall. The debris is then collected and removed by the catheter.

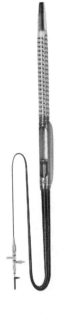

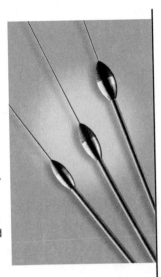

Figure 13.
Rotational
Atherectomy
Device
This diamond-encrusted, olive-shaped device, called the Rotablator® rotational atherectomy system, rotates at high speed to remove hard, calcified blockages.

ing plaque (see Figure 13). Rotational atherectomy may be particularly useful for removing large quantities of plaque and very long or very hard blockages.

If you are having rotational atherectomy, you may need a temporary pacemaker inserted before your angioplasty.

Thrombectomy Devices

A blood clot (**thrombus**) is common in coronary arteries of patients with severe or recent angina, or those who are having a heart attack (see Figure 1, page 3). Sometimes a thrombus can form during the angioplasty procedure itself, increasing the risk of a heart attack and other long- and short-term complications. To reduce this risk, your physician may use a **thrombectomy device** before he or she inserts an angioplasty balloon and stent. Currently, these devices effectively remove blood clots by suction, although their long-term benefits have yet to be proven in clinical studies. New devices in development (see Figure 14) use a cutting device in addition to suction, to break up the clot before removal. Thrombectomy may be more uncomfortable than ballon angioplasty because larger guiding catheters are used.

Figure 14. Thrombectomy Device

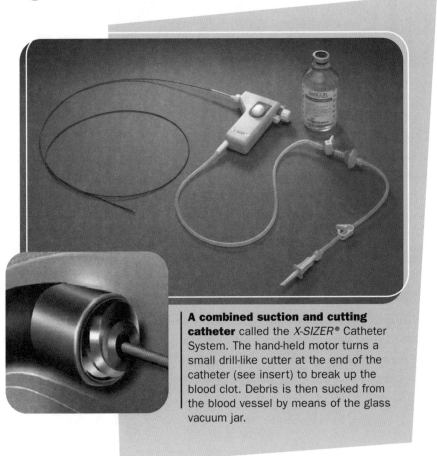

A combined suction and cutting catheter called the *X-SIZER®* Catheter System. The hand-held motor turns a small drill-like cutter at the end of the catheter (see insert) to break up the blood clot. Debris is then sucked from the blood vessel by means of the glass vacuum jar.

Laser Devices

Various laser devices have been tested in the treatment of angina with little or no success. Lasers have been incorporated into balloons to try to improve angioplasty results and onto the tips of angioplasty guide wires to help them pass through blocked blood vessels. To date, no studies have demonstrated the advantages of any laser device in any situation. Most laser devices are now gathering dust in the corners of cath labs.

Additional (Adjunctive) Techniques and Devices

In addition to the techniques available to treat narrowed or blocked blood vessels, several devices can be used to help improve their long-term results.

Intravascular Ultrasound

The use of ultrasound in general (using sound waves bounced off part of the body to form an image) has had a huge impact in all fields of medicine. It is used to diagnose disease, to check the health of an unborn baby, and as a treatment. You may have had a cardiac ultrasound to assess the strength of your heart muscle or the function of your heart valves.

An ultrasound probe (which sends and receives sound waves to build up a picture of your heart) can now be miniaturized and inserted into blood vessels in a procedure called intravascular ultrasound (IVUS). This is normally performed as part of an angioplasty, or is occasionally done during an angiogram. It provides more accurate images of your blood vessels than angiography does (see Figure 15). A recent study has shown that arteries are less likely to re-narrow if IVUS is used to guide the placement of a stent. IVUS is currently used in fewer than 5 percent of all Canadian angioplasty procedures, but its use is increasing slowly.

Figure 15. The inside of a coronary artery, as revealed by IVUS (intravascular ultrasound)

IVUS provides a more accurate picture of an artery, including the central space (the lumen), the wall, and any blockages (plaque). By comparison, a coronary angiogram only reveals the lumen.

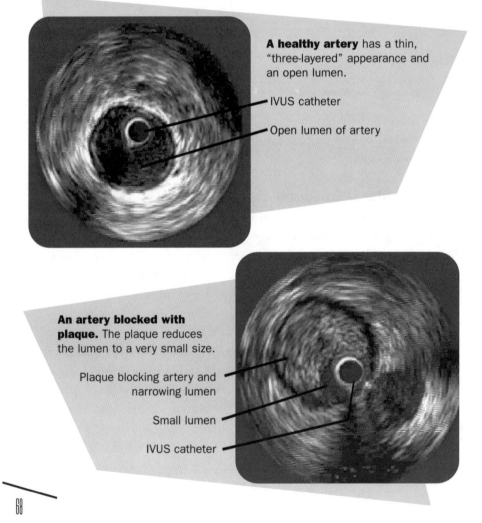

A healthy artery has a thin, "three-layered" appearance and an open lumen.

IVUS catheter

Open lumen of artery

An artery blocked with plaque. The plaque reduces the lumen to a very small size.

Plaque blocking artery and narrowing lumen

Small lumen

IVUS catheter

Doppler Flow Wire

A Doppler flow wire uses ultrasound to measure the actual blood flow down coronary arteries, in the same way that radar guns are used by traffic police to measure the speed of vehicles. The ultrasound device is mounted onto the end of a very small wire, similar to the angioplasty guide wire.

Blood flow in healthy arteries increases by a factor of three during exercise. In the cath lab, a short-acting drug is usually given to simulate exercise. The Doppler flow wire is then used to decide whether an angioplasty is required or when it has been successful. The Doppler flow wire may not give accurate results for people with diabetes or high blood pressure.

Pressure Wire

This device is similar to the Doppler flow wire, but instead of using sound waves to measure blood flow, the pressure wire measures the drop in pressure across the blockage. In normal or mildly narrowed blood vessels, there is only a small drop in pressure (less than 25 percent) inside a blood vessel during exercise. As with the Doppler flow wire, a drug is used to simulate exercise and the pressure wire then measures the degree of blockage before and after angioplasty.

What Happens Next?

Everyone is different, and technology moves fast, so if you have any questions about the techniques that your physician may use in your particular case, be sure to discuss them with him or her before your angioplasty procedure.

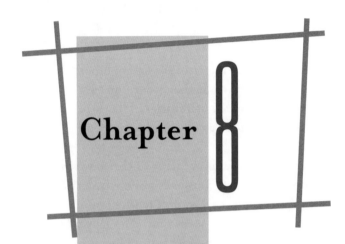

Chapter 8

when it's all over

What Happens in this Chapter

- The immediate aftermath
- Your return to the ward
- Symptoms to watch for
- Care of your wound
- Eating and drinking
- Going home checklist

After your angioplasty you will spend a few hours recovering. You will need to stay in bed, lying flat while your puncture closes. Nursing staff will keep an eye on you overnight to check that all is well. You will then be allowed to go home.

Bed rest

As soon as your angioplasty has finished, you will be transferred —still flat on your back—to a recovery area or directly back to the ward. If you have had your angioplasty via your groin, you will not be allowed to sit up for several hours. You may find this uncomfortable and difficult to tolerate, particularly if your angioplasty procedure took a long time, but there are some good reasons for it. The amount of sedative and the effect it has varies from patient to patient, but the medical and nursing staff will want to make sure that you are no longer groggy before you get out of bed. There is also a risk of bleeding or bruising if you sit up in bed or get out of bed too early since angioplasty involves a puncture in a major artery. Moreover, your blood is "thinner" from the blood-thinning drugs for your angioplasty.

[S E L F - H E L P]

Back problems

Backache is a particularly common complaint from many patients after angioplasty and can make the recovery period even more uncomfortable. If you have back problems, tell your physician BEFORE you go into the cath lab.

If you suffer from back problems, or have any orthopedic complaints that may prevent you from lying comfortably in bed for a few hours after your angioplasty, you must tell your physician *before* your procedure. He or she has several options to reduce the amount of time you spend lying down afterward, and to minimize your discomfort. These include the use of closure devices to seal the blood vessel in your groin immediately after your angioplasty (see page 60) or the use of the blood vessel in your wrist for your angioplasty, instead of your groin (see page 61). Neither of the above options is available to you or your physician once you leave the cath lab, so be warned!

Arrival Back on the Ward

After your angioplasty your medical team will do everything they can to ensure that you have a safe recovery. To prevent problems from arising, or to ensure that any problems are dealt with quickly, the nursing staff will take a number of precautions upon your arrival in the ward or recovery area:

- The nurse accompanying you from the cath lab will give a short report to the ward or recovery area nurse. This will normally include a brief summary of your angioplasty, the drugs given to you in the cath lab, additional drugs that may be needed after your procedure, and any problems that occurred during your angioplasty. He or she will also mention specific problems for your nurse to watch for.

- You will be asked if you have any symptoms such as chest pain or breathlessness. Don't try to be "brave." If you have any symptoms, mention them right away.

- The site of the puncture will be checked regularly for signs of bleeding or bruising because your blood will be thin for the first few hours after your angioplasty.

- A blood sample will be taken for routine testing.

- ECG electrodes and wires will be attached to your chest and legs to connect you to a heart monitor.

- A routine ECG will be performed.

- Your "vital signs" (heart rate and blood pressure) will be checked regularly. This may involve the use of an automatic blood pressure machine pre-set to measure your blood pressure every few minutes after you arrive on the ward. Blood pressure and heart rate checks will become less frequent as time goes on.

- Your intravenous lines will be checked to ensure that they are running properly and that the correct dose is being delivered to you.

> "They gave me painkillers when we left the operating room because I asked. Whatever I wanted in terms of pain relief, they gave me."
>
> **Arni Cohn**

Friends and Family

After your angioplasty, friends and family will no doubt be anxious to know how you are and to hear about what happened. You may also be keen to speak to them. However, your safety comes first. Before you have visitors, the nursing and medical staff need to check your condition and carry out the safety procedures listed above. Once these have been performed and your condition has been confirmed as stable and satisfactory, your family will be allowed to see you.

What If I Get Chest Pain?

You may experience slight chest pain or discomfort at the end of your angioplasty. Your physician will try to prevent this or treat it while you are in the cath lab, but this may not be possible, in which case you will leave the cath lab with some left-over chest discomfort. This usually improves gradually over the next few minutes or hours.

The most likely reason for pain after an otherwise successful angioplasty is blockage of one or more of the tiny blood vessels that branch off the main blood vessel dilated by the balloon. If your medical team identifies this as the cause of your lingering chest pain, they will give you a pain-relieving injection. You should still tell your nurse if the pain increases or does not improve over time.

If you have no pain when you leave the cath lab, but start to develop chest pain afterwards, your medical team will check you over carefully before you are given pain medication. Your heart rate and blood pressure will be measured and, possibly, a new ECG taken. What happens next will depend on what the tests show. If your chest pain continues, you may simply be given nitroglycerine under your tongue or a strong pain-relieving drug such as morphine. In the unlikely event that your chest pain is due to re-narrowing or blockage of your blood vessel, you will need to be taken back to the cath lab for a repeat coronary angiogram and, possibly, a further angioplasty.

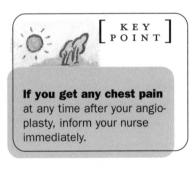

[**KEY POINT**]

If you get any chest pain at any time after your angioplasty, inform your nurse immediately.

Blood Tests

Blood tests will be done routinely after your angioplasty.

Very infrequently, the number of platelets in the blood (**blood count**) can fall as a side effect of all the blood-thinning drugs and injections involved in the angioplasty procedure. Having an adequate blood count is important because platelets help blood to clot. If your blood count does fall, you will be at risk of bleeding from your groin until the wound fully heals (see below). As a matter of routine, your blood count will also be re-checked the day after your procedure and before you are discharged from the hospital.

Your blood will also be tested to check for damage to your heart. Sensitive blood tests are now available, called **troponin tests**, that can detect even the slightest damage. Using such tests, recent studies have shown that some people suffer very small heart attacks during or after angioplasty that would otherwise go undetected. Although physicians are still debating whether these very small heart attacks are significant, if your troponin test comes out positive you may need to stay in the hospital a little longer and have some further tests as a precaution.

"I can remember my body tilting when they put the pressure on the one side. It's very uncomfortable and there's a certain amount of indignity when you have to go to the bathroom, but that's to be expected...it's like having your tooth out and saying, 'Well, I've got to eat soup the next couple of days.' It just kind-of goes with the procedure. And after the one day—you're done."

Bill Hogarth

Care of Your Wound

Once you return to the ward, the nursing staff will check the site of your puncture or wound frequently. You should also be aware of how you feel and keep a look out for symptoms such as bleeding, swelling, or pain. Let your nurse know immediately if anything is bothering you. What happens next with your puncture depends on how your angioplasty was performed.

Late Sheath Removal

If your angioplasty was performed via your groin, your physician may leave the sheath in place for a few hours after your angioplasty, held in place by a small stitch (**suture**) or tie. This is the traditional approach and is done to allow the effect of the blood-thinning drugs to wear off a bit before your sheath is removed to reduce the chances of bleeding or bruising. It also allows a repeat angioplasty to be performed quickly if the blood vessel re-narrows or blocks anytime after your procedure.

If the sheath is left in place, you will be kept flat on your back in bed for 4 to 6 hours before it can be removed. *You will not be able to bend your leg—even for a moment—because the sheath will bend inside the artery and cut off the blood supply to your leg.*

The exact amount of time the sheath stays in your groin can vary from hospital to hospital. It can also depend on the results of your blood tests. Once your sheath is removed, you will have to stay in bed for a further 4 to 6 hours, still lying completely flat. Your nurse may place a sandbag or clamp on your groin to provide extra pressure. Overall, with this method, you will be in bed for about 10 to 12 hours, and occasionally longer.

To remove your sheath, your medical team will give you a local anesthetic injection and then snip the suture holding the sheath in place. The sheath will then be pulled from your groin in a way similar to the way it was done after your angiogram and a clamp or manual pressure will be applied to the area for 15 to 30 minutes to prevent bleeding. Sheath removal may be a little uncomfortable, but is not usually painful.

Once the sheath is out and there is no sign of bleeding, the manual pressure will be released or the clamp removed. Nursing staff will continue to keep an eye on you in case of further bleeding.

Closure Devices for Your Groin

One of the alternatives to prolonged bed rest is the use of closure devices (see page 60), which can halve the time you need to spend in bed. If you have a closure device, you won't be allowed out of bed immediately, but you may be able to sit up in bed shortly after your arrival back on your ward and, assuming that all is well, be allowed out of bed after 4 to 6 hours. You may need to lie flat for much of this time. As with a sheath, your closure device will be checked at regular intervals and, if you become aware of any bleeding, you should let your nurse know.

Angioplasty Via your Wrist

If your angioplasty has been performed via your wrist, the sheath is removed immediately and replaced by a small clamp or tight bandage to stop any bleeding. When this has been done, you can sit up in bed right away. You may even be transferred to your ward in a wheelchair rather than a bed. There is some bed rest, but much less than with groin angioplasty, and you will be able to get out of bed within a few hours.

"The sheath came out sometime in the afternoon, although I can't remember it very well. There is no pain, the only discomfort is afterwards, when you can't move."

Mrs. C.V.

11

Once back on the ward after your wrist angioplasty, your nurse will check your wrist at regular intervals for bruising, swelling, or bleeding. The bandage or clamp on your wrist is normally removed after 1 to 2 hours and replaced with a small adhesive bandage.

Eating and Drinking

"It's strange when you're on your back and they bring you lunch... eating sandwiches lying down isn't easy."

Bill Hogarth

There are two main limitations to eating and drinking after angioplasty. First, it is difficult to eat and drink while you are lying flat in bed. Second, food and drink are normally delayed for a few hours after your angioplasty as a precaution in case any complications develop. In the unlikely event that your blood vessel did re-narrow or block in the first few hours after your angioplasty, you may need to have another angioplasty or, possibly, an emergency bypass operation. So even though you will be hungry, you will still need to wait a few hours after your angioplasty before eating and drinking. Once this precautionary period is over, you should be able to eat and drink normally.

Same-Day Discharge

The number of days that patients spend in the hospital after an angioplasty has fallen over the years because angioplasty techniques have improved. You will probably only spend one night in the hospital after your angioplasty before being discharged, although this will depend on the severity of your heart problems and how well you recover from the angioplasty. Some hospitals in Europe are starting to send patients with successful angioplasties home later the same day and angioplasty is viewed as just another day surgery or minor surgical procedure. We may see this happening in Canadian hospitals in the near future.

Pre-Discharge Consultation

Before you are officially discharged, you will normally be seen by your angioplasty physician or nurse for a pre-discharge consultation. Now is the time to ask all your questions. You will obviously want to know how successful your angioplasty was, and what are the chances of your angina returning in the future. You will also want to know what to do in the event of an emergency. Once you have asked your questions, your physician or nurse will have lots of advice and information for you (some of this will be covered in Chapter 9). It is often a good idea to have a friend or relative present at this time simply as another pair of ears. Try writing things down, as well, to help you remember what you have been told.

Leaving the Hospital

Before you rush out of the hospital you might find the following checklist useful, to make sure that you have everything you need.

CHECKLIST – LEAVING THE HOSPITAL   ✔

- Letter to your family doctor   ◯

- Prescription for your "stent tablets" or other new drugs   ◯

- Contact name & number in case of emergency   ◯

- General information package (groin care, etc.)
  including a list of dos & don'ts   ◯

- Someone to escort you home   ◯

- Follow-up appointment (if applicable)   ◯

- Your personal items   ◯

- This book!   ◯

What Happens Next?

Once you are discharged you can go home, relax, and concentrate on making your recovery.

Chapter 9

recovering at home

What Happens in this Chapter

- Dealing with medication
- Care of your wound (at home)
- What to do in an emergency
- Guidelines for getting back to work
- Exercise, sex, driving, and flying
- Follow-up visits to your doctor or clinic

The first few days after your angioplasty can feel like an uphill struggle. Your incision may hurt and you may be wondering whether you'll ever feel healthy again. By following a few simple guidelines and gradually increasing your activity, you will find that life soon starts to feel more normal. By 6 months after your procedure, you should know whether your angioplasty was successful.

Your First Day Back Home

ONCE YOU GET OUT OF THE HOSPITAL, DON'T OVERDO THINGS. GIVE your body time to adjust. Everyone is different so there are no absolute rules—except listen to your own body and do things within your own limits. Here is a useful list to remind you what you should, and should not, be doing.

[KEY POINT]

DO...	DON'T...
Take it easy	Rush back to work
Get plenty of sleep	Do any heavy lifting or strenuous exercise
Start a "heart healthy" diet	Assume that since your angioplasty was successful, you can now return to your previous unhealthy diet and heart-unhealthy habits
Plan an exercise routine	Forget that your groin will take 10 full days to heal
Try some self-help techniques, such as relaxation or massage	Forget to take your medication
Try to keep stress to a minimum	Allow yourself to get stressed
Quit smoking	Continue to smoke

For advice on diet, exercise, and relaxation, see Chapter 10

Changes to Your Medication

Your medication may or may not be changed after your angioplasty, depending on your health and the physician who treats you. Some physicians may reduce your angina medication immediately after a successful angioplasty because your angina is greatly improved. More commonly, your medication is not changed until your first visit to your cardiologist or family doctor approximately 1 month after your angioplasty. He or she may then decide to reduce your medication based on a number of factors (see More Detail box).

Don't be surprised if you leave the hospital on more medications than you were on when you

> "I didn't let my heart problems stop me from doing what I wanted, but I'm cautious. If I feel any signs, I listen carefully to my body. All heart patients should learn to be in tune with their body."
>
> **Arni Cohn**

Which Pills? 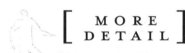 [**MORE DETAIL**]

After your angioplasty, your physician will prescribe long-term medication based on the following factors:

- How you feel
- How quickly you return to normal
- Whether you need medication for other medical conditions, for example, high blood pressure
- Your cardiac risk factors
- Whether you had a stent inserted into your blood vessel
- The type of stent inserted into your blood vessel

arrived. If you had a stent inserted into your blood vessel during your angioplasty, you will definitely be sent home on either clopidogrel (Plavix) or ticlopidine (Ticlid) in addition to your other medications (see page 45). You will stay on these "stent drugs" for 1 to 6 months.

Your cardiologist may also decide that you are not taking enough medicine to stop your heart disease from getting worse. He or she may start you on medicine to reduce your blood cholesterol, lower your blood pressure, and help with heart failure, or, if you were on these medications before, the dose may be increased.

It is important that any physician who treats you knows about *all* the medications that you are on—not just drugs for your heart, but all medicines—including those that you buy over the counter without a prescription (for instance, herbal remedies, supplements, drugstore pain relievers). As the number of drugs you take increases, so do the chances of side effects from interactions between them. Remember that even complementary remedies such as herbal medicines have drug-like effects on your body and may interact with medicines that your doctor has prescribed for you, so be sure to tell him or her about them. You may find the diary pages at the back of this book useful for keeping a record of your medications.

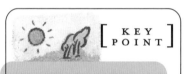

[KEY POINT]

Make sure you know
exactly what medicines you should be taking and that you have a sufficient supply of tablets to take when you get home. You may wish to add your new medication to the diary pages of this book.

Caring for Your Incision

Your groin (or wrist) will be checked one last time before you leave the hospital. It is a good idea to take a shower rather than a bath on the first day after your angioplasty to reduce the risk of your groin or wrist starting to bleed again. It is worthwhile checking your groin or wrist for signs of oozing or swelling every now and again, especially if you start to feel any pain in the area. Be prepared for a small amount of bruising. This is more common after angioplasty than angiography because of the blood-thinning drugs that you received during your angioplasty. It is sometimes difficult to decide between normal bruising and bruising that needs medical attention. In general, contact your doctor for any bruise associated with swelling or pain (rather than just simple discomfort).

Physical Activity

It is normal to expect some discomfort from the site of your incision because your blood vessel will take 7 to 10 days to heal completely. If you had angioplasty via your groin, you should avoid strenuous exercise and heavy lifting for a week or two. If you have a physically demanding job, this may be a major inconvenience, but it pays to be careful at this stage because a return visit to the hospital as a result of bleeding would be even more inconvenient. If you had your angioplasty via your wrist, you do not need to be as careful, but you may feel discomfort if you do activities that put strain on your wrist, such as tennis, golf, or gardening.

Once your incision site has healed, regular exercise should be your top priority. Exercise is an essential part of your recovery and is one of the best therapies for your heart. It's a good idea to set goals for yourself and you might find it helpful to actually write them down (for instance, in the diary at the back of this book). Try to include exercise in your everyday routines. Walk up stairs instead of taking the elevator. Walk to the corner store or park (or gym) instead of using the car. Even when you are sitting down watching television, you can still do exercises such as leg lifts. Gradually, you will build up your stamina and, with a sensible exercise program, you should be able to achieve more and more—and feel better and better.

Pain or Breathlessness— What Do You Do?

If at any time you start to feel pain, short of breath, or your chest starts to feel "tight" STOP WHAT YOU ARE DOING IMMEDIATELY. It is NOT normal to experience breathlessness, central chest pain, or pain radiating down your left arm. If your pain does not go away, go to your nearest Emergency Room or call 911. This is just a precaution, in case your coronary artery suddenly blocks after you leave the hospital.

When you leave the hospital, your information package will include a telephone number for you to contact for help or advice regarding any other problems or questions you may have.

> "The night after I got home I couldn't get my breath, like a panic attack, so I went back to the hospital. The doctor decided it was just that the arteries were sensitive and throbbing or pulsating, giving the breathless feeling. I had an angiogram later on and everything was fine."
>
> **Bill Hogarth**

Sexual Activity

Once at home you can quickly resume a normal sex life, although it's a good idea to take it easy for the first few weeks. It is not uncommon to feel very uneasy about resuming a normal sex life with your partner, especially if you have had a heart attack. In fact, sexual intercourse isn't as hard on your heart as you may think. The Heart and Stroke Foundation of Canada calculates that the effort required is roughly equivalent to walking up two flights of stairs. General advice is to resume lovemaking when both you and your partner feel ready. You may find the American Heart Association guidelines helpful (see More Detail box).

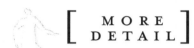

Affairs of the Heart
—Sex After a Heart Attack

[**MORE DETAIL**]

The American Heart Association gives the following suggestions for lovemaking after a heart attack. These tips are also useful for people with angina.

- Choose a time when you are rested, relaxed, and free from stress brought on by the day's schedules and responsibilities.
- Wait 1 to 3 hours after a meal to allow it to digest.
- Select a familiar, quiet setting where you are unlikely to be interrupted.
- Take medicine before sexual activity, if prescribed by the doctor.
- Take it easy. Allow adequate time for foreplay, both to get your heart going gradually and to recapture some intimacy after spending time apart.

If you experience a rapid heartbeat or have difficulty breathing for 20 or 30 minutes after intercourse, have angina pain, or feel very tired the next day, consider slowing the pace down a bit.

In time, the partner who has had a heart attack or heart surgery is usually able to resume the same activity level as before (if not more so).

Driving

There is no law against driving immediately after your angioplasty, but most hospitals will recommend that you allow time for your groin to heal. In Canada the rule of thumb is that you can start to drive 2 to 3 days after your angioplasty, although your physician may suggest a longer or shorter wait.

Flying

The recommendations on how soon after your angioplasty you can fly are determined more by medical insurance companies than by physicians. Although you will probably be able to sit comfortably after a couple of weeks, you may find it difficult to get travel health insurance until 3 months, and sometimes up to 6 months, after your angioplasty.

"Of course it's in the back of your mind when you go on holiday somewhere—especially to the States."

Robert (Bobby) Frew

Returning to Work

If you have a sedentary job, you can return to work very quickly after your angioplasty. If your work involves either strenuous exercise or heavy lifting, you should wait at least 10 full days before going back to work to reduce the risk of triggering angina and, if you had angioplasty via your groin, to allow your groin to heal. If you have a *very* strenuous job (a firefighter, for example), it may be wise for you to be checked out by your family doctor or cardiologist before you return to work. He or she may wish to send you for a **treadmill test** (see Glossary) to assess your cardiac condition before giving you the "all clear."

Visits to Your Physician

The hospital will probably recommend that you visit your own cardiologist or family doctor 4 to 6 weeks after your angioplasty. The reason for this is to allow him or her to check that you are generally well, to examine your groin (or wrist), and perhaps to confirm that it is safe for you to return to work, if you're still off. You may also need a repeat prescription for any new medications prescribed to you following your angioplasty. Since the "stent drugs" clopidogrel and ticlopidine are usually prescribed for only 4 weeks you may be taken off these medications at this stage. If you are well, and free of angina, the number of medicines you are taking may be reduced.

There are no essential tests needed after your angioplasty, apart from the blood tests for ticlopidine (see below). If your physician does recommend any tests, these will be similar to the ones you had before your angioplasty. Your cardiologist may ask you to do a treadmill test at around 1 month after your angioplasty, with or without a **nuclear perfusion scan** (see Glossary).

If you are discharged from the hospital on ticlopidine, you will be asked to visit your family doctor every week for a routine blood test. This is just a precaution because ticlopidine can occasionally affect your bone marrow, causing your white blood count to fall.

The number of times you need to visit your cardiologist or family doctor after your first visit depends on how you are and on your doctor's preference.

Follow-up Clinic Visits

The physician who performed your angioplasty may wish to see you for one or more follow-up appointments. This may not happen for a while if your own cardiologist or family doctor is sending in reports of your progress. Since your blood vessel can re-narrow (or **re-stenose**) within the first 6 months, the cardiologist who performed your angioplasty may make your first appointment 6 months after your angioplasty when this "danger period" has passed. At this point, he or she will tie up any loose ends with you and discuss your future. If your symptoms of angina have returned, this meeting is useful for organizing a further treadmill test, a repeat angiogram, and a further angioplasty, if needed. If you are feeling well, don't expect to be offered a further angiogram to "prove" that your angioplasty worked. Most cardiologists in Canada are guided by their patients' symptoms: if you don't have any angina symptoms, you are unlikely to undergo any more testing, unless (like our patient Mr. Hogarth) you are part of a clinical trial.

"When I went back for my second angiogram, my 6-month check-up, stress test. and blood work, and they said it was all fine and I could resume a normal life....What a mental high!"

Bill Hogarth

Beyond 6 Months

If you are well 6 months after your angioplasty, your return visits to your cardiologist or family doctor should become less frequent. Unless you have other medical problems, you will only need to see your physician one or twice a year for routine follow-up. The emphasis now changes from looking after your symptoms to trying to prevent future problems.

What Happens Next?

Once you have recovered from your angioplasty and things have returned to normal, you will, we hope, feel better than ever before. It's important to realize, though, that your heart disease has not been cured. Your angioplasty has only bought you time—time to take stock of your life, time to realize that your heart is in your hands. If you want to change your life, the next chapter shows you how.

how you can help yourself

What Happens in this Chapter

- Lifestyle shifts that can transform your future
- Changing your diet—the simple and easy way
- Exercising your way forward
- Supplements and herbal medicines
- Massage, visualization, acupuncture, relaxation
- The science of complementary therapies

It is a common misconception that angioplasty is a cure for heart disease and that it removes the disease from your coronary arteries. In fact, neither angioplasty nor heart bypass surgery stops your heart disease from gradually getting worse. That part is up to you. Just as a combination of factors contributed to your heart disease, a combination of treatments is the only effective way forward. This includes a long-term commitment to exercise, dietary changes, and quitting smoking. Correcting only some of your risk factors, while ignoring others, will not work.

Healing Your (Whole) Self

IN THIS CHAPTER WE WILL LOOK AT WAYS IN WHICH YOU CAN improve your heart health through exercise and diet. We will also explore techniques such as visualization and relaxation and other complementary therapies that you can use to help you prepare for your angioplasty procedure and take control of your life afterwards.

Most of the therapies mentioned use a holistic approach to your health. The word "holistic" comes from the Greek word *holos* meaning "whole." Holistic health care involves treating the whole person and not just one isolated body part or one risk factor. When you are considering what you can do to help yourself, think of healing your whole self and not just your heart.

[S E L F - H E L P]

Help Yourself to a Healthy Heart

The "big four" (M.E.D.S.)

- **M**anage stress
- **E**xercise
- **D**iet
- **S**moking (stop)

Some people also find these approaches helpful:

- Vitamins and supplements
- Herbal medicines
- Visualization and relaxation techniques
- Massage, therapeutic touch, and acupuncture

Healthy Lifestyle and Heart Disease

The old adage "you are what you eat" holds a great deal of truth, particularly when it comes to heart disease. Heart disease is a disease of over-fed countries. It is important to take a step back, take a good look at your diet, and plan out what improvements you should make.

Many studies have shown that healthy eating can stop your heart disease from getting worse and, in combination with exercise and weight loss, may even reverse it. However, it must be a long-term commitment. Improving your diet for only a short period of time will make no difference to the health of your heart because athero-sclerosis—the artery-hardening process that causes heart disease—is a chronic (long-term), not an acute (short-term), disease.

Changing the eating habits of a lifetime can be hard, especially if you aren't very confident in the kitchen. Most hospitals can refer you to a cardiac rehabilitation program or dietitian, who will give you plenty of encouragement and practical advice.

What Is a "Heart Healthy" Diet?

Healthy eating involves eating a well-balanced diet containing foods from all the main food groups. No one food group alone can provide you with all the necessary nutrients needed to maintain health.

> "You have to drive the recovery and rehabilitation exercise. I went on a 9-month program designed to change your lifestyle and work you hard. The idea was a permanent change, to select a different road. I saw tremendous denial by other participants who thought they could cheat a bit."
>
> **Arni Cohn**

Fruit and Vegetables

There is plenty of evidence to show that a diet rich in fruit and vegetables helps to protect against and, potentially, reverse cardio-vascular disease. Fresh fruit and vegetables are high in nutrients and fiber and low in calories. The exact reasons why they protect against heart disease is unknown. Part of the reason may be that a diet rich in high-fiber foods is likely to contain less saturated fat, a major cause of heart disease (and obesity, another risk factor for heart dis-ease). It is also likely that there are active ingredients within fresh fruit and vegetables that help the body fight disease, including heart disease. The active ingredients are unknown, so beware of expensive supplements in health food shops that claim to be full of them. Try to eat at least 5 servings of fruit and vegetables each day and, if pos-sible, eat organic produce and what is currently in season because these will be fresher and contain more nutrients.

Fiber

Most of us don't eat enough fiber, so it makes sense to boost this important part of your diet. This should help to reduce your cho-lesterol level and, because fiber fills you up without adding calories, it will also help to reduce your calorie intake and lower your body weight. You can get more fiber by incorporating plenty of fresh fruits and vegetables, as well as whole grains, nuts, and cereals (oatmeal, wheat germ, whole oats, etc.) into your diet.

"You have to work at it. Exercising, losing weight, changing diet, it's hard. A posi-tive attitude is the best thing."

Robert (Bobby) Frew

Fats

When you're trying to choose heart-healthy food it can get pretty confusing trying to sort out what you're meant to be doing about those fats. Dietitians now keep the advice simple: reduce your fat intake overall and *especially reduce saturated fats*. The easiest rule of thumb for managing this is to avoid products high in animal fats—all those hamburgers and hot dogs. The reason for this is that most animal fat is saturated fat.

If you wish to eat dairy produce, try to stick with the lower-fat or non-fat products. These would include skim or 1 to 2 percent fat milks, low-fat yogurt, and low-fat cheeses. Try using polyunsaturated or monounsaturated margarines for spreading on baked potatoes, bread, or other baked goods, and olive or canola oils for dressings, sauces, and frying.

How Low Do You Go?

There is a scientific debate raging, particularly in the U.S., over whether very low-fat diets (containing around 10 percent of calories from fat) can actually reverse heart disease. Some studies appear to support this idea, while others seem to show that once you get down to a certain point (about 25 percent), there is no further benefit gained from reducing fat. The debate will no doubt continue to get more interesting, but in the meantime, the advice in Canada is to aim for about 30 percent of calories from fats (many people find that hard enough), and reduce saturated fats and trans fats.

> "Don't kill yourself if you don't follow-through 100 percent. Just try harder next time round."
>
> **Arni Cohn**

Protein Sources

Use a variety of protein sources such as fish, soy products, lean meat, poultry, and legumes. If you do eat meat, stick to lean cuts and small portions. There is good evidence to show that eating at least one portion of oily fish per week (such as mackerel and sardines) has a heart-protective role in coronary heart disease (see page 104, "Omega-3 fatty acids").

Beans, nuts, and legumes are great sources of protein and thus can be used as an alternative to fatty meats, as can soy products. Nuts and seeds also contain polyunsaturated fats (the "good" fats).

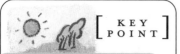

[KEY POINT]

Diets are hard, so let's keep the rules simple. Eat much more fiber, fruit, and vegetables and significantly reduce your total fat intake, especially saturated fats.

Salt

It is a good idea for all heart patients to limit their salt intake. Prepared foods, processed foods, and take-out type foods are generally high in salt. The current recommendation is less than 3 grams of salt per day—about half a teaspoon.

Alcohol

Alcohol can be a pleasant part of a social occasion, but it can also be harmful for people with heart disease. Studies show that men who drink more than 20 alcoholic drinks per week are at an increased risk of both stroke and raised blood pressure (see More Detail box). Alcohol is also extremely high in calories and thus contributes to weight gain. If you have raised triglyceride levels in your blood, you should avoid alcohol completely. Some heart medications should not be combined with alcohol: it is best to check with your pharmacist if you are unsure.

The issue of whether alcohol has a protective effect on your heart is controversial. The idea is called the "French paradox"—named after the image of the French nation as being heart-healthy, despite their love of high-fat food, due to a lifetime of wine-drinking. How

What is a Drink? 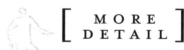 **[MORE DETAIL]**

Canadian guidelines on healthy alcohol consumption suggest that women should have no more than one drink, and men no more than two, per day.

1 drink = 5 oz glass of wine = 1 bottle of beer = 1.5 oz liquor

true this image of the French nation is, remains to be proven, as does the French paradox itself. Some studies suggest that, in very small amounts, alcohol may protect against coronary heart disease and stroke. However, when the risks and benefits are taken into consideration, the bottom line is that if you don't drink at present, you should certainly not *start* drinking with the hope that you may protect yourself against heart disease.

Help Yourself to a Healthy Diet

The following are some tips to help you eat your way to health:

- Take a heart-healthy cooking course. It will be fun, you'll meet other people in the same position as you, and you'll learn how food can be delicious as well as healthy.

- Load up on fruit, vegetables, and fiber at every meal. That way you'll have less room for fatty foods.

- Try to use broths instead of gravy.

- If you eat meat, each portion should be no bigger than the palm of your hand.

- Watch those "low-fat" bakery and dessert items. They are often very high in sugar, so you'll put on weight—which is also bad for your heart.

- Be aware of hidden saturated fats. Not all food labels list the saturated fat content. Be particularly suspicious of baked goods and pre-prepared meals.

- Avoid deep-fried foods. They are usually high in saturated fat or they may have a lot of **trans fats** (hydrogenated vegetable oils), the worst kind of fat for your heart.

Check Your Weight

It's hard, we know it is, but if you have heart disease, achieving and maintaining a healthy body weight is essential. Weight gain is associated with an increased risk of coronary artery disease and stroke. If you lose weight you may also reduce your blood pressure. The more gradual your weight loss, the greater the chance that the weight will stay off. "Crash diets" are an unsafe way to diet and, in the majority of cases, the weight will be regained. A consultation with a registered dietitian can help you work out what your ideal weight should be and help you set goals to achieve it. Keeping to the healthy diet guidelines above may be all that is needed to shed the extra pounds.

Check Your Blood Pressure

High blood pressure is the "silent killer" because it usually has no symptoms but makes your heart disease worse. If you have heart disease, you will almost certainly be taking blood-pressure-lowering medication, but you can further reduce your blood pressure with lifestyle modifications, in particular, losing some weight and reducing your salt intake.

Check Your Cholesterol

The most important thing you can do to lower your cholesterol, in addition to taking your cholesterol-lowering medicine, is to reduce the amount of saturated fat that you eat. There is also some evidence that soluble fiber, found in foods such as oatmeal, can lower blood-cholesterol levels.

[S E L F - H E L P]

Use the diary pages of this book to record and track your lifestyle goals. You can also use them to keep track of all your medications, including complementary medications.

Cigarette Smoking

There is overwhelming evidence that smoking is, without question, disastrous for the health of your heart. The good news is that it is never too late to stop. Your risk of a heart attack or death falls rapidly once you stop smoking—by as much as 40 percent, according to one study. There is advice and support available to help you give it up. Talk to your GP, cardiologist, or nearest cardiac rehabilitation program.

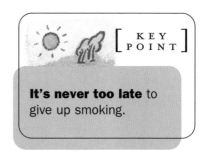

[KEY POINT]

It's never too late to give up smoking.

Exercise

We all know about it, we've all done it (some of us still do it), not many of us do enough of it, and we all know how good it is for us.

Exercise is essential. There are no alternatives to it and you alone are responsible for doing it, since no one can do it for you. Exercise can play a huge role in your recovery and long-term well-being. It can help you lose weight, it may lower your blood pressure, and may even stimulate new blood vessels to grow in your heart. Choose a sensible exercise program that suits you. The general guidelines in Canada recommend that adults should do 30 minutes of moderate exercise at least 5 days of the week. Moderate activities are cycling, fast walking, swimming, or heavy-duty housework.

"With exercise I became normotensive for years. I learned to walk at a proper pace so as not to stress myself. I now walk a minimum of 6 hours a week. If I walk more I don't get credit for it, but if I walk less I have to make up for it next week."

T. Hofmann

Get a Helping Hand

We strongly recommend that you enrol in a cardiac rehabilitation program, which will give you specific targets to aim for, general support, help, and advice based on your individual needs.

Stress Management

Our lives today contain enormous amounts of stress. Stress is the body's "fight or flight" response with nowhere to go, so the burden that stress places upon the body is huge. It acts as a silent and slow-acting body debilitator—almost like a disease in itself when it is left unattended. It can be years before we realize just how much stress we are under. It can take years, again, to actually recognize that we need to do something about it. Even if we try to ignore stress, our bodies are extraordinarily clever at giving us warning signs that we are over-doing things. It is essential that you learn to recognize these signs and do something about them.

Following are a few ideas that you might like to consider to control or manage your stress. See also Relaxation, Meditation, and Massage (pages 106–108).

"During the day I sit down for 2 or 3 minutes and internalize to see if I'm doing okay. If I've gone 2 or 3 hours without doing that, I know it mentally—I stop and relax and pull back, take a couple of deep breaths and say, 'How am I feeling?'"

Arni Cohn

Go for a Walk

You may not feel like it at the time, but once you get outside a walk can do wonders for clearing your head and lowering your blood pressure.

Deep Breathe

Sit down somewhere quiet (even if it means sitting in the washroom), and inhale and exhale slowly and deeply. As you breathe out, try to imagine all your anger or frustrations being blown out with your breath. Say to yourself, "I do not need this stress, my health is more important." Repeat this to yourself a few times before you go back to what you were doing.

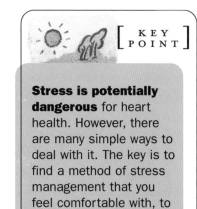

[KEY POINT]

Stress is potentially dangerous for heart health. However, there are many simple ways to deal with it. The key is to find a method of stress management that you feel comfortable with, to provide relief for your heart (and your head!).

Try to Avoid Arguments and Conflict

Avoiding a fight may be easier said than done, but nothing raises the blood pressure more effectively than a heated argument. Once again, ask yourself if the issue that is making you angry or frustrated is more important than your health. Is it possible to wait a few minutes or hours when all those involved in the conflict have calmed down? Perhaps then the issue at hand can be discussed more rationally and quietly.

Get Plenty of Sleep

Lack of sleep can only add to the stresses of the day. You can improve your chances of a good night's rest by
- not having caffeine after 4pm
- going to bed at the same time every night
- trying to sleep only when you're tired
- having a comfortable mattress
- buying some earplugs if your partner snores

Find a Hobby

Outdoor hobbies such as gardening are particularly helpful for stress. They can re-focus your mind and stop you from thinking about things that make you feel stressed.

Take Your Watch Off

Our lives are ruled by time. How many times in a day do you look at a clock or a watch? Find a day when you have nothing planned, take your watch off, and spend the day doing what you want, according to how you feel. Eat when you are hungry, rest when you feel tired, and fill in the rest of the time your way. You will be amazed at how re-energizing this can be.

Vitamins and Supplements

If you eat a well balanced diet (see above), it should provide you with all the essential nutrients and vitamins you need to achieve optimum health. You should consider vitamins and supplements only if you are not able to maintain a well-balanced diet.

If you have ever walked into a store selling vitamins and dietary supplements you will know that it can be overwhelming and confusing. If you are considering taking a supplement, seek out a professional such as a dietitian, qualified nutritionist, or naturopathic doctor who can recommend what you need to best complement your diet.

Multivitamins

Studies have shown that high doses of multivitamins can be unhealthy for heart disease patients. If you are considering multivitamins, consult a qualified professional.

Vitamins C and E (the antioxidant vitamins)

Despite many scientific studies, there is still no clear-cut evidence that vitamin C and E supplements make any difference one way or another to heart disease patients. It seems that vitamin E at a dose of 100 to 400IU daily, combined with a diet high in fruits and vegetables and plenty of exercise, *may* be beneficial in heart disease patients. For vitamin C, there is still no overwhelming evidence that it is beneficial as a treatment for heart disease when taken as a supplement. In fact, the Los Angeles Atherosclerosis Study recently showed that high doses of vitamin C (850mg to 5,000 mg/day) may make matters worse. This study found that artery disease progressed *faster* in patients taking these high doses of vitamin C, than it did in patients who did not take vitamin C supplements.

So why did some studies show a benefit and others did not? One possible explanation of why the vitamin supplements were ineffective in some of the studies is that the patients were sticking to a healthy diet and receiving adequate vitamin C and E anyway, so the supplements were unnecessary.

[**KEY POINT**]

It is *essential* to inform all people involved in your care what supplements and medicines you are taking to avoid the risk of dangerous drug interactions. Physicians need to know about all non-prescription medicines and supplements; complementary therapists need to know about prescription drugs.

Folic Acid, B6, and B12

There has been a lot of interest in these supplements as a treatment for heart disease because deficiencies in these vitamins can cause high blood levels of an amino acid, linked to cardiovascular disease, called **homocysteine**. However, there is not, as yet, evidence to show that these supplements prevent or reverse atherosclerosis. A better choice might be simply to eat more fruit and fresh vegetables.

Co-enzyme Q10

Co-enzyme Q10 is a naturally occurring enzyme found within the body tissues, particularly in the heart, liver, and pancreas. To date, there have been no substantial studies on humans to prove its benefit for treating heart disease when given as a supplement (despite what the Internet may tell you).

Omega-3 Fatty Acids

Omega-3 fatty acids have been shown to have a protective role in coronary heart disease. To obtain your omega-3s without supplements, eat at least one fatty-fish meal per week or incorporate flax seeds, flaxseed oil, canola oil, and nuts into your diet.

Herbs

Herbs have been used as medicines since the beginning of humankind, and many of today's prescription medicines are based on natural substances found in herbs. Although there are numerous herbs advocated for use in heart disease, clinical studies have only been carried out on a few. Hawthorn has the most overwhelming evidence that it works.

Hawthorn

In large, well-designed clinical studies similar to those carried out on prescription drugs, hawthorn has been shown to increase blood flow to the coronary arteries, strengthen the heartbeat, and decrease blood pressure. It also has antioxidant properties and minimal side effects. Hawthorn is widely used throughout Europe as a medicine for the heart, often in combination with conventional drugs. However, hawthorn can affect the blood levels of other drugs, such as digitalis, glycosides, beta-blockers, and other blood-pressure-lowering drugs.

Garlic

There is good scientific evidence that garlic can protect your heart. One study, published in the *Journal of the Royal College of Physicians and Surgeons of London* in 1994, showed that eating 1/2 to 1 clove of garlic per day can reduce cholesterol levels by as much as 12 percent. Other reputable studies have shown that it has a blood-thinning effect, by reducing the stickiness of platelets (see Glossary), and can reduce the stiffness of the main blood vessel of the body, the aorta, in elderly people.

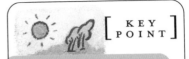

[**KEY POINT**]

Because of the blood-thinning effect of garlic, you should stop taking it (either raw or in capsules) at least 10 days prior to your surgery or you may be more susceptible to bleeding. If you are thinking of starting garlic capsules and you are already taking other blood-thinning medications, talk to your physician.

Ginko Biloba

Ginko is not as well-researched as hawthorn and garlic, but there are a few studies that show it increases blow flow and is an effective treatment for some circulatory diseases. A recent review of all studies, published in the *American Journal of Medicine* in 2000, concluded that ginko is particularly beneficial for treating artery disease in the blood vessels of the legs.

Other Herbs for Heart Disease

Other herbs used to treat cardiovascular disease for which there is scientific evidence include Terminalia arjuna, a traditional Ayurverdic herb used for heart conditions since the sixth century B.C., and tumeric. A recent study published in the *International Journal of Cardiolology* showed that Terminalia arjuna has benefits for patients with heart failure. Tumeric appears to have anti-platelet, cholesterol-lowering, and antioxidant properties.

The following herbs have been traditionally used to lower blood pressure, although there are no reputable scientific studies to either prove or disprove their effectiveness: olive leaves, cramp bark, yarrow, dandelion leaves, lime flowers, and mistletoe.

Safety Note

It must be *strongly* advised that if you are considering exploring the use of herbs to assist you with your health you consult an experienced herbalist or naturopathic doctor. Herbs and prescription drugs can interact, with serious side effects.

Other Complementary Therapies

Relaxation

It is widely recognized within the medical profession that people who learn to relax can control symptoms and, in some cases, even reduce blood pressure or pain. Relaxation can be achieved in a number of ways, including meditation, yoga, deep breathing, a nice hot bath, or simply imagining yourself lying on a hot, sunny beach. The trick is finding ways to relax in your current anxious state. Many cardiac rehabilitation programs now teach relaxation techniques as an integral part of recovery and there are numerous tapes and books on relaxation, so check out your local bookstore.

Meditation

Sit in a quiet place, focus on your breathing, and find a word or phrase that you can say over and over again to yourself. For example, you might try phrases that rid you of negative feeling towards other people and help you to accept personal differences. Letting go of such destructive feelings will give you more energy to focus on your own health and well-being. You might also consider a meditation program such as Tai Chi.

Visualization

This is a form of meditation that involves using mental imagery to bring about the changes you wish for. The idea—a visual version of "positive thinking," which may explain its apparent success in some people—is to believe that the more clearly you can see your desired future, the more chances there are of it becoming true. An example would be to imagine your blocked artery, unblocked. Although your angioplasty will accomplish this, positive thinking may, indeed, help your long-term health. There are numerous studies showing the power of the mind in medicine. Visualization can be practiced alone or in groups, and it usually requires the help of a therapist or tapes.

Acupuncture

Acupuncture has been in use for over 3,500 years in China and involves inserting fine needles into the skin and underlying tissues. Acupuncture practitioners consider acupuncture to work by stimulating the "vital force" or *qi* (pronounced chee)—the spiritual, mental, emotional, and physical aspects of a person. Although science has neither proven nor disproven that acupuncture works this way, what we do know is that it can relieve angina and anginal-type symptoms in some people.

Massage

Massage is the art of using the hands to stimulate the skin and muscles to bring about a feeling of comfort and to promote healing. The Bible, the Qur'an, and the Ayur-Veda all mention the use of

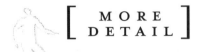
Complementary therapies for heart disease are, *generally speaking*, not as widely researched as conventional drugs or surgeries and the studies that do exist are often not up to the standard of conventional drug trials. This means that we don't always know about side effects or how people with different diseases might be affected, so be cautious. A therapy isn't safe just because it's "natural" (the natural world contains some of our most powerful poisons). There are, however, a surprising number of good studies and the science of complementary therapies always makes for fascinating reading. See "Resources" at the back of this book.

massage. There are many forms of massage, including Swedish, shiatsu, aromatherapy, reflexology, and neuromuscular. It can be a very positive experience and is the perfect way to reduce stress.

Chelation Therapy—Does It Work?

Chelation therapy has been in use for approximately 40 years in North America for many different chronic illnesses. Heart disease patients generally receive chelation therapy intravenously (into a blood vessel). The theory is that chelation agents improve circulation by removing undesirable elements such as calcium and toxic metals from the blood, thus helping to reduce disease in the walls of blood vessels.

Intravenous chelation therapy in heart disease is extremely expensive and there are *no* reliable clinical trials proving that it works. If you are considering chelation therapy you should think about it carefully, given the potential for adverse side effects, the expense, and the lack of any documented benefit.

What Happens Next?

If you have heart disease, no drug or surgery will work by itself. Likewise, no complementary therapy should be considered an "alternative" therapy, that is, a replacement for medical intervention. A combination approach—medical therapy, diet, exercise, other complementary approaches—is going to give you the best chance of slowing your heart disease and, possibly, even reversing it. Be sure to always tell your doctor about any complementary treatment that you decide to undertake. Likewise, be sure to tell any complementary practitioner about your angioplasty.

"It's best to be realistic. I have accepted that some things I won't change, and I've tried to work on everything else."

Arni Cohn

   You are now well equipped to take full control of your heart's health. In the next chapter we look at the long-term results of angioplasty and how you can decide whether the procedure worked for you.

Chapter 11

has my angioplasty worked?

What Happens in this Chapter

- How you might feel right away
- What you might expect as you recover from the procedure
- The long-term picture

The success of your angioplasty procedure will usually be judged by how you feel, both immediately afterward and in the 6 months that follow. The majority of patients find that angioplasty relieves most or all of their angina symptoms and that they have no long-term problems.

Immediate Results

PATIENTS DO NOT LEAVE THE CARDIAC CATHETERIZATION LABORATORY until the angioplasty has finished and the physician has achieved the best possible result. You will therefore know fairly quickly how successful your angioplasty has been. If your physician is busy after your procedure and is not able to discuss the results with you right away, the cath lab nurses often will.

The Recovery Period

Once you have arrived back on the ward or recovery bay, your nurses will repeatedly ask how you are and encourage you to report any symptoms of chest pain immediately. If you have no chest pain, you can assume that your procedure is, thus far, a success.

Exactly how much better you feel when you are out of bed and walking around will depend on the severity of your angina symptoms before your angioplasty. If your angina was previously brought on by very little exercise, then you should notice an immediate improvement. If your symptoms were moderate in severity beforehand, for example, needing a brisk walk to bring on the pain, you will probably not notice any difference until you leave the hospital. If your angina was mild before the procedure, that is, brought on only by vigorous exercise, then you may have to wait some time before knowing how well your angina has responded to the angioplasty. This is because you will not be able to exercise until your groin has fully healed.

"It was interesting because they took a photo from the video screen before and after so I could see the blockage, then see it being cleared. It's a positively uplifting thing to see that."

Bill Hogarth

Partial Revascularization

In some patients it is not technically possible, or it is too risky, to remove all the blockages in the coronary arteries. This result is known as **partial revascularization**, in contrast to **total revascularization** where all the narrowings are successfully treated. If this is true in your case, you may be told that your angioplasty has been successful on the blood vessels that were treated, but that it was not possible to deal with all the narrowings. Disappointing, perhaps, but you should still gain some benefit. Although you may still have angina, you may find that you can tolerate more exercise before symptoms start.

In the rare cases where a physician attempts angioplasty, but is not successful (for whatever reason), obviously the symptoms of angina will remain unchanged.

> "The main difference afterwards was how often the angina happened, and how bad it was. It used to be really bad, four or five attacks daily, but now I just get it occasionally or if I forget to put on the patch. I do get tired more easily, but that's normal for getting older."
>
> **Mrs. C.V.**

The First 6 Months

Once you leave the hospital, your doctor will judge the success of your angioplasty mainly on *how you feel*. This may sound pretty untechnical, but studies have shown that using hospital tests to monitor the response to angioplasty is usually no more helpful than just asking the patient about his or her symptoms.

The first 6 months are crucial because this is the window during which re-narrowing (or **re-stenosis**) of your coronary arteries happens, if it is going to. Studies show that one-third of patients have some re-stenosis, so re-narrowing of the arteries can almost be considered normal. However, the important consideration for each patient is whether this means that angina symptoms return. This so-called "clinical re-stenosis" happens in 10 to 20 percent of patients who have had a stent inserted, and 20 to 30 percent of patients after balloon angioplasty alone. If you are unlucky and this does happen to you, your original symptoms of angina will return.

> "If you're out of surgery, you're not dead. Don't sit there morose. Take a deep breath, look around, and say, 'You know what? I'm here now. I feel better, I have an opportunity. Let me get ahead with it.'"
>
> **Arni Cohn**

What Happens Next?

If you experience angina at any stage after this 6 months, it is probably due to narrowing in one of your other coronary arteries as your heart disease progresses. This is why it is important to understand the reasons that you developed angina in the first place and do your best to make lifestyle changes to improve your heart's health.

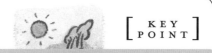

[**KEY POINT**]

If you do not correct your "cardiac risk factors," such as smoking, obesity, lack of exercise, and a high-fat diet, your other blood vessels may become blocked in the future.

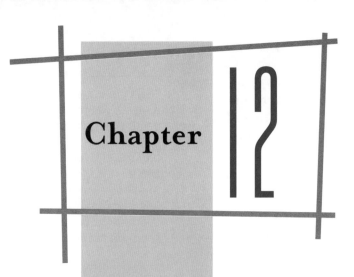

Chapter 12

medications

What Happens in this Chapter

- The major medications for angina
- How they work and the main side effects
- How to find the right medication mix for you

You are the most important member of your own care team, and never more so than when it comes to medications. You should always understand why you are taking each medicine, how to take it correctly, and any possible side effects, so that you can help your physician find the best combination for you. Medications for treating angina include medicines to prevent your angina symptoms and to treat them when they do arise, and drugs to stop your heart disease from getting worse.

What Drugs Do You Need?

IF YOU HAVE ANGINA, YOU HAVE PROBABLY BEEN prescribed several kinds of medicines. They have three purposes:

- To prevent (or at least reduce) the number of angina attacks that you have (beta-blockers, calcium channel blockers, and nitrates).

- To treat angina attacks if and when they occur (nitrates).

- To prevent the disease in your blood vessels from becoming worse (anti-platelet agents, anticoagulants, lipid-lowering drugs, and anti-hypertensives).

The precise types and doses of drugs that your doctor has prescribed for you to prevent or treat your angina depend on how severe your symptoms are, whether you suffer from any other illnesses, and how likely you are to experience the side effects of a particular drug.

Drugs that prevent your heart disease from getting worse are needed because neither angioplasty nor bypass surgery actually stops the progress of the disease. Therefore, even if you undergo angioplasty or bypass surgery, you will need to take one or more of these "preventive" drugs afterward—possibly for many years in the future. The full list of medications your physician will prescribe depends on many factors, including whether you have had a heart attack, have high blood pressure, or have some other heart problem.

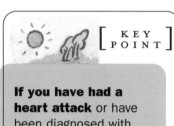

[**KEY POINT**]

If you have had a heart attack or have been diagnosed with heart disease, it is likely that you will remain on some drugs for the rest of your life. It is quite possible to become almost drug free if you are prepared to make dramatic lifestyle changes, but you may still be advised to keep taking ASA (Aspirin).

All too often, patients just take what their doctor prescribes without question. It is important that you understand why you are taking medication and what it is for. It also helps to know its possible side effects, so that you are able to recognize them if they occur and tell your doctor, who may be able to change your medication. By having a clear understanding of your medications, you can also provide your doctor with an accurate report of how well your drugs are working. It may take more than one try to find the medication or combination of medications that works best for you.

What's in a Name?

The various names given to drugs can be confusing and frustrating. Not only does every drug have at least two names, there is often more than one kind of any particular drug. For example, nitroglycerin spray is the same drug no matter who makes it, but it is marketed under many different names. The brand that you will use generally depends on your doctor's preference, drug cost, or the hospital's policy.

The two names that every drug has are the **generic name** and the **brand** or **trade name**. The generic name is the non-trade name for the drug molecule. This is the official drug name that has been approved by regulatory authorities worldwide and it never changes. This way, safety information on the drug can easily be tracked throughout its life. The brand or trade name is the proprietary or copyright name that is given to the drug by its manufacturer. This is usually different in different countries.

When a drug is first developed, its manufacturer has an exclusive right to manufacture and market it for a number of years. This right is called a patent and usually means that the drug is known by only one brand name. Once the patent expires, other manufacturers are allowed to make the drug and may give it a number of different brand names. This is why drugs with different names may have exactly the same active ingredients (although the non-active ingredients, like colorings, may differ).

Drugs for Angina

All drugs are classified into groups based on what they do and how they work. There are hundreds of drugs that treat diseases of the heart and blood vessels (so-called **cardiovascular drugs**). Drugs that you are likely to be given can be divided into the following groups:

Nitrates

Nitrates, such as nitroglycerin, are used to both prevent and treat angina attacks. They have been in use for more than 75 years. Nitrates widen blood vessels, thereby increasing blood supply to the tissues (including the heart muscle) and reducing the amount of work the heart needs to do.

Beta-Blockers

These drugs reduce blood pressure, heart rate, and the strength of the heart's contraction. As a result, the heart needs less oxygen. Beta-blockers have been used for more than 20 years.

Calcium Channel Blockers

Also called **calcium antagonists** or **CCBs**, these drugs relax the muscles around blood vessels, thus widening arteries and increasing the blood flow and oxygen delivery to the heart muscle. They have been available since the 1980s.

Angiotensin-Converting Enzyme (ACE) Inhibitors

ACE inhibitors are a relatively new class of drugs, mainly used to treat high blood pressure and heart failure. However, they have also been shown to prevent angina from getting worse, to prevent heart attacks and severe angina, and to strengthen the heart muscle after a heart attack. They block the production of a substance that constricts blood vessels, thereby widening blood vessels and increasing the amount of oxygen that gets to the heart.

Anti-Platelet Agents

Once a blood vessel is narrowed by atherosclerosis, a blood clot can form on the blockage, causing severe angina or a heart attack. Anti-platelet agents reduce the tendency of blood platelets to form blood clots. There are a number of different ones (see Medications Table) with different uses, depending on how potent they are. ASA (Aspirin) is a useful anti-platelet agent that can be taken every day. Angioplasty greatly increases the risk of blood clots, so just before your angioplasty you will be given a stronger anti-platelet agent such as clopidogrel (Plavix). During the procedure itself, when the risks are greatest, you may be given a highly potent anti-platelet therapy through your vein, such as abciximab (ReoPro), one of a group of drugs called **glycoprotein IIb/IIa inhibitors**. (For more on these drugs, see page 52.)

Anticoagulants

Anticoagulants also prevent blood from clotting through a different mechanism from the anti-platelet agents. You can take anticoagulants as preventive medicine, for example, warfarin (Coumadin), or be given one (such as heparin) during your angioplasty.

Lipid-Lowering Drugs

Lipid-lowering drugs reduce the level of cholesterol and other fats in the blood. This helps to prevent your heart disease from getting worse by slowing down or stopping further narrowing of your coronary arteries.

Other Blood-Pressure-Lowering Drugs

Beta-blockers, calcium channel blockers, and ACE inhibitors (see above) all reduce blood pressure in addition to their benefits for angina. Other types of blood-pressure-lowering drugs, or **anti-hypertensives**, that you may be prescribed include the **diuretics** ("water pills") and **angiotensin-II receptor antagonists** (**ARBs**, for short).

Drugs Used in the Treatment of Angina

This table includes both generic names and trade names, in alphabetical order, so you can look up either one.

Generic Name, *Trade Name*	Drug Class
abciximab, *ReoPro®*	anti-platelet agent
Accupril™, **quinapril**	ACE inhibitor
acebutolol, *Monitan®, Sectral®*	beta-blocker
acetylsalicylic acid (ASA), *Aspirin®*	anti-platelet agent
Adalat®, **nifedipine**	calcium channel blocker
Aggrastat™, **tirofiban**	anti-platelet agent
Altace®, **ramipril**	ACE inhibitor
amlodipine, *Norvasc™*	calcium channel blocker
Aspirin®, **acetylsalicylic acid (ASA)**	anti-platelet agent
ASA (acetylsalicylic acid), *Aspirin®*	anti-platelet agent
atenolol, *Tenormin®*	beta-blocker
benazepril, *Lotensin®*	ACE inhibitor
Betaloc®, **metoprolol**	beta-blocker
Capoten™, **captopril**	ACE inhibitor
captopril, *Capoten™*	ACE inhibitor
Cardene®, **nicardipine**	calcium channel blocker
Cardizem®, **diltiazem**	calcium channel blocker
Cedocard®, **isosorbide dinitrate**	nitrate
Chronovera®, **verapamil**	calcium channel blocker
cilazapril, *Inhibace®*	ACE inhibitor
clopidogrel, *Plavix™*	anti-platelet agent
Corgard®, **nadolol**	beta-blocker
Coumadin®, **warfarin**	anticoagulant
diltiazem, *Cardizem®, Tiazac®*	calcium channel blocker
enalapril, *Vasotec®*	ACE inhibitor
eptifibatide, *Integrilin®*	anti-platelet agent

felodipine, *Plendil®, Renedil®*	calcium channel blocker
fosinopril, *Monopril™*	ACE inhibitor
Hepalean®, **heparin**	anticoagulant
heparin, *Hepalean®*	anticoagulant
Imdur®, **isosorbide-5-mononitrate**	nitrate
Inderal®, **propranolol**	beta-blocker
Inhibace®, **cilazapril**	ACE inhibitor
Integrilin®, **eptifibatide**	anti-platelet agent
ISMO®, **isosorbide-5-mononitrate**	nitrate
Isoptin®, **verapamil**	calcium channel blocker
Isordil®, **isosorbide dinitrate**	nitrate
isosorbide dinitrate, *Cedocard®, Coronex®, Isordil®*	nitrate
isosorbide-5-mononitrate, *Imdur®, ISMO®*	nitrate
labetalol, *Trandate®*	beta-blocker
lisinopril, *Prinivil®, Zestril®*	ACE inhibitor
Lopresor®, **metoprolol**	beta-blocker
Lotensin®, **benazepril**	ACE inhibitor
metoprolol, *Betaloc®, Lopresor®*	beta-blocker
Minitran®, **nitroglycerin**	nitrate
Monitan®, **acebutolol**	beta-blocker
Monopril™, **fosinopril**	ACE inhibitor
nadolol, *Corgard®*	beta-blocker
nicardipine, *Cardene®*	calcium channel blocker
nifedipine, *Adalat®*	calcium channel blocker
Nitro-Dur®, **nitroglycerin**	nitrate
nitroglycerin, *Minitran®, Nitro-Dur®, Nitrol®,* *Nitrolingual®, Nitrong®, Nitrostat™,* *Transderm-Nitro®, Tridil®*	nitrate
Nitrol®, **nitroglycerin**	nitrate
Nitrolingual®, **nitroglycerin**	nitrate
Nitrong®, **nitroglycerin**	nitrate
Nitrostat™, **nitroglycerin**	nitrate
Norvasc™, **amlodipine**	calcium channel blocker
pindolol, *Visken®*	beta-blocker
Plavix™, **clopidogrel**	anti-platelet agent
Plendil®, **felodipine**	calcium channel blocker
Prinivil®, **lisinopril**	ACE inhibitor
propranolol, *Inderal®*	beta-blocker
quinapril, *Accupril™*	ACE inhibitor
ramipril, *Altace®*	ACE inhibitor

Renedil®, **felodipine**	calcium channel blocker
ReoPro®, **abciximab**	anti-platelet agent
Sectral®, **acebutolol**	beta-blocker
Tenormin®, **atenolol**	beta-blocker
Tiazac®, **diltiazem**	calcium channel blocker
Ticlid®, **ticlopidine**	anti-platelet agent
ticlopidine, *Ticlid®*	anti-platelet agent
timolol, *Blocadren®*	beta-blocker
tirofiban, *Aggrastat™*	anti-platelet agent
Trandate®, **labetalol**	beta-blocker
Transderm-Nitro®, **nitroglycerin**	nitrate
Vasotec®, **enalapril**	ACE inhibitor
verapamil, *Chronovera®, Isoptin®, Verelan®*	calcium channel blocker
Verelan®, **verapamil**	calcium channel blocker
Visken®, **pindolol**	beta-blocker
warfarin, *Coumadin®*	anticoagulant
Zestril®, **lisinopril**	ACE inhibitor

The trade names of these drugs are based on information available at the time of publication. They may change. If in doubt, look for the generic name on your box of medication.

What About Side Effects?

All drugs have the potential to cause side effects. The goal is to avoid side affects or keep them to a minimum so that you don't notice them too much and they don't do any harm. Read the information that comes with your drugs or ask your pharmacist or physician about the possible side effects of your medication.

Potential Side Effects of Angina Medications

Drug Class	Common side effects
ACE inhibitors	cough, low blood pressure, headache, dizziness, tiredness, nausea or vomiting, kidney problems, rash, altered sense of taste, swollen ankles, fever, joint pain
Anticoagulants	stomach pain, hair loss, blurred vision, rash, hives, itching, loss of appetite, diarrhea, skin discoloration, bruising
Anti-platelet agents	dizziness, chest or stomach pain, headache, rash, diarrhea, vomiting, flushing, swollen ankles, joint pain
Beta-blockers	contraction of the throat muscles, tiredness, dizziness, low blood pressure, sleep disturbances, slow heart rate, cold hands and feet, diarrhea, constipation, nausea or vomiting, impotence, skin discoloration, fever
Calcium channel blockers	headache, fast or slow heart rate, stomach upset, constipation, swollen tissues, dizziness, urinary frequency, palpitations, low blood pressure, flushing, tiredness, insomnia, muscle stiffness
Nitrates	dizziness, fainting, headache, low blood pressure, irregular heart rhythms, nausea, blurred vision, sweating

Help Yourself to the Right Medications

- Always take your medication exactly as prescribed.
- Be sure to document any side effects that you may be experiencing and inform your physician immediately. Do not suffer unnecessarily.
- Keep a list of the drugs that you have taken in the past in case a doctor or nurse needs to know about your use of a specific medication.
- You can use the diary pages of this book to record which medications you are taking, what they are for, any changes in your medication, and any side effects you are experiencing.

What Happens Next?

When you leave your doctor's office with a prescription, the next steps are up to you. Surprising as it may seem, many people with life-threatening conditions do not fill their prescriptions and when they do, often fail to take the medication properly—or at all. Your medicines are part of your recovery process, so be sure to take them exactly as prescribed. Don't forget, too, that if you make lifestyle changes to improve your health, your doctor may be able to reduce the number or dose of medications that you take (see Chapter 10 for some help with this).

Chapter 13

the future of angioplasty

What Happens in this Chapter

- Taking part in a clinical trial
- Up-coming tools and techniques that could further improve the results of angioplasty

Patients already benefit from the technological strides that angioplasty has made in the last two decades. However, the procedure still has its limitations, so the quest for new and better techniques continues. Up-coming tech-nologies that may soon become realities for patients include stents that patch tears in arteries, self-absorbing, radioactive, and drug-coated stents, and devices to break up and remove blockages.

Clinical Trials and You

WHEN YOU ARE ADMITTED TO THE HOSPITAL FOR YOUR ANGIOPLASTY, you may be asked to take part in a research trial for a new angioplasty technology or a new drug for use during angioplasty procedures. Because Canadian hospitals have a worldwide reputation for excellence in conducting clinical research trials, there are many such studies ongoing in Canada.

If you are approached, carefully read the documents the research nurse (see Chapter 14) will give to you before agreeing to anything. If you agree to take part, you will need to sign a written consent form. If you have any questions or want any more details before you sign, ask your physician or the research nurse before your procedure. If you still have lingering doubts about being involved, don't be afraid to say no. It will not count against you: your physician will continue to provide you with the care that is right for you.

> "I was in a study, so I went back afterwards and had another angiogram. It showed no problems at all. No bruising, and no problems with the procedure outcome."
>
> **Bill Hogarth**

Less is More: Trends in Angioplasty

The advances that have been made in angioplasty over recent years are part of a general trend for surgical procedures to be performed through smaller and smaller incisions. This increase in **key-hole** or **minimally invasive surgery** has been driven by patients and hospital administrators, as well as by physicians. Patients generally prefer minimally invasive surgery because the scalpel incisions leave smaller scars and allow for a quicker recovery. Hospital administrators also like minimally invasive surgery because it lets patients leave the hospital (and free up bed space) earlier.

Angioplasty—being a minimally invasive technique—has always had the advantage over bypass surgery in that it involves less patient trauma, a faster discharge from the hospital, and a quicker recovery. Because of these advantages, angioplasty technology is here to stay and will continue to develop. The goal of angioplasty research is, first, to enable physicians to get better results by gradually overcoming some of the limitations of angioplasty (see page 30). The second goal is to help patients who are not currently suitable for angioplasty, such as patients with blockages that have been present for many years.

Recent Improvements in Angioplasty

The routine use of stents during angioplasty has improved both the short- and long-term results of the procedure. Emergency bypass surgery following angioplasty, which is usually needed if the blood vessel becomes blocked after the angioplasty balloon is inflated, has now fallen from as much as 3 percent to less than 1 percent of all procedures. The long-term picture has also improved: studies show that the risk of re-stenosis (with a return of your angina) after stent insertion is only 10 to 20 percent, as opposed to 20 to 30 percent with balloon angioplasty alone.

Furthermore, improvements in both the design and construction materials of angioplasty equipment have significantly improved the performance of catheters, guide wires, balloons, and stents—and made them easier for physicians to use.

Finally, new blood-thinning drugs (see page 52) have reduced the frequency of blood-clotting problems and the occurrence of small heart attacks during angioplasty, without increasing the risk of major bleeding complications.

Drug-Coated Stents

This area is probably *the* hottest topic in angioplasty today. The hope is that drug-coated stents will solve the number one problem with angioplasty: the high rate of re-narrowing. A variety of drug-coated stents are currently under investigation. Their aim is to prevent, or reduce, the scar formation that occurs inside stents, which reduces the open space in the blood vessel (lumen) and the flow of blood. Side effects for the patient are unlikely because the drug only goes to where it is needed. However, these stents are still in development and none is available for use yet.

Radioactive Stents

In many diseases, radiation treatment is used successfully to reduce excessive scar tissue. In the hope that this technology may also benefit angioplasty patients, studies have been going on for many years using radioactive stents.

Like drug-covered stents, the aim of radioactive stents is to reduce the amount of scar tissue.

The results have been somewhat disappointing so far. Getting the correct dose of radiation onto each stent has been difficult. There is also an ongoing risk that dangerous blood clots will form on these stents (a condition called **thrombosis**) because they do not become coated with the normal lining of the blood vessel, unlike conventional stents.

Covered Stents

Stents lined with a membrane made of Teflon were originally designed for angioplasty of heart bypass grafts. The plaques in this type of bypass graft crumble much more easily than in the heart's natural arteries, so there is a greater risk that portions of the plaque may fall away during the angioplasty procedure, block a blood vessel downstream, and cause a heart attack. Membrane-covered stents hold the plaque in place as the stent expands, preventing debris from escaping (see Figure 16).

Covered stents are also increasingly being used for angioplasty of the heart's own arteries, although they are not suitable for all blood vessels. These stents can help strengthen blood vessels with weak walls (**aneurysms**) and are useful for the emergency treatment of blood vessels that tear during the procedure.

Figure 16. A covered stent

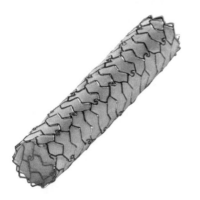

This special stent is, in fact, two stents with Teflon material sandwiched in-between. It is designed to reduce the risk of stray pieces of plaque blocking blood vessels downstream.

Self-Absorbing Stents

Self-absorbing stents slowly dissolve into a blood vessel after their insertion. These devices may improve the long-term results of stenting. They may also allow future bypass surgeries to be performed more easily because there is no metal meshwork to get in the way of the new bypass grafts. It is an interesting idea and a potentially exciting development for the future. However, there is only one self-absorbing stent currently under investigation and its long-term results are not yet known.

Brachytherapy

Brachytherapy is another way of using radiation to try to prevent re-narrowing after angioplasty (see Figure 17). It may prove to be the best way to deal with stents that have re-narrowed along their entire lengths. However, there is no evidence so far that brachytherapy prevents re-narrowing in arteries *without stents*. It also means additional exposure to radiation and a longer, more complicated procedure that requires the combined skills of a cardiologist and a radiation oncologist (cancer specialist).

Figure 17. Brachytherapy Device

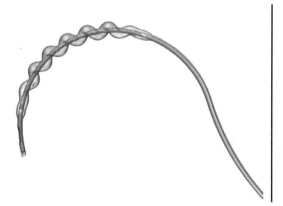

This spiral-like balloon, called the GALILEO™ Centering Catheter, uses radiation to reduce the re-narrowing of stents. The radioactive material is on the tip of a wire that is inserted into the center of the balloon. The spiral balloon may allow blood to flow down the artery while applying radiation equally throughout the artery's length and width.

Electro-Mechanical Mapping

This state-of-the-art technology is currently useful as a research tool to measure the effectiveness of different treatments. It involves inserting a sensor into the main pumping chamber of the heart (the left ventricle).

It is the only technology available that can exactly measure both the electrical and mechanical condition of the heart muscle. The downside is that there is a small risk of damage to the heart muscle. It is also not yet clear what role (if any) it might play in hospitals, although it may help angioplasty physicians and cardiac surgeons decide whether or not to operate on particular areas of the heart after a heart attack.

Cutting Balloon™ Device

The Cutting Balloon device is similar to an ordinary angioplasty balloon, but it allows the blockage to be pushed against the artery wall more easily (see Figure 18). This means that it can open blockages with much lower pressure than a conventional balloon and, therefore, reduces the injury to the artery wall. Some studies show that it also reduces the rate of re-narrowing. Cutting Balloon devices may prove to be especially beneficial for blockages at the entrance of a blood vessel or inside a stent.

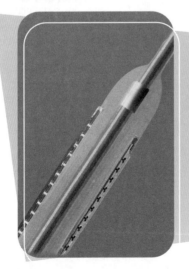

Figure 18.
Cutting Balloon™ Device
This angioplasty balloon has three or four blades attached to the outside that cut into the hard blockage when the balloon is inflated. This makes the artery wall less rigid and easier to stretch.

Distal Protection Devices

In some types of blood vessels and blockages, when the angioplasty balloon inflates, pieces of plaque fall off and get carried downstream, where they block smaller arteries. This is called **distal embolization**, and can result in a slowing or stopping of your heartbeat, angina, or even a heart attack.

Distal embolization is more common in angioplasty of bypass grafts and where the narrowed part of the artery contains a blood clot. To prevent distal embolization in these types of narrowings, specially designed catheters can be used to catch the debris before it gets swept away. Two different types of devices are currently under development (see Figures 19 and 20).

If the early promise of these devices is confirmed, they may be used routinely during angioplasty of bypass grafts and carotid arteries, and in people who have had a heart attack.

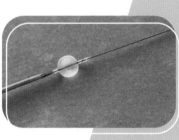

Figure 19.
PercuSurge™ Device
The special balloon is positioned beyond the blockage before the angioplasty balloon is inflated. Any debris that falls from the artery wall is trapped within the vessel, since there is no flow, and removed by the suction tube.

Figure 20.
FilterWire™ Device
This tiny funnel-shaped filter acts like a fishing net to catch any debris released from the plaque during balloon angioplasty.

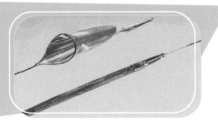

Chapter 14

who's who of hospital staff

What Happens in this Chapter

- Hospital staff you will meet
- A brief overview of their roles

When YOU GO INTO THE HOSPITAL, YOU WILL ENCOUNTER A LARGE
number of staff. Generally speaking, the hospital staff will be
friendly and approachable. If you are dealing with them directly,
they should introduce themselves and explain their role in your
care. However, sometimes they are busy and unable to take the time
to tell you how they can help you during your hospital stay.

To add to the confusion, many of the hospital staff, from porters
to doctors, wear white coats or "scrubs" (loose pants and tops),
making it hard to figure out who's who. In addition, within the title
of "doctor" or "nurse" are a number of different roles, making it
difficult to work out what each of these people do. For example, you
may see a "fellow," a "resident," or a "staff physician." All are doctors, but all have varying levels of knowledge and ability. Or, you
may see a ward nurse, an angioplasty nurse, a nurse practitioner,
and/or a research nurse. Again, all are qualified nurses, each with a
different role.

This chapter will give you a brief overview that explains who is who
in the hospital and what each person does.

[**MORE DETAIL**]

Medical Staff	**Nursing Staff**	**Ancillary/Support Staff**
Staff cardiologist	Ward nurse	
Fellow	Nurse practitioner	Nursing assistant
Resident	Cath lab nurse	Ward clerk/recep-
Medical student	PTCA nurse	tionist
	Research nurse	ECG technician
		Blood technician

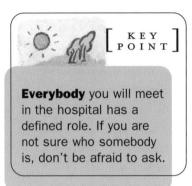

[KEY POINT]

Everybody you will meet in the hospital has a defined role. If you are not sure who somebody is, don't be afraid to ask.

Ward Clerk / Receptionist

Usually the first person you will meet upon your arrival to the ward. He or she is responsible for organizing the administration of the ward. Often his or her role extends beyond this, depending on experience level.

Ward Nurse

A qualified nurse who works on the ward providing patient care. These nurses have a range of roles depending on seniority and experience. They are responsible for your well-being and safety during your stay on the ward.

Nurse Practitioner

A qualified nurse who has usually completed a masters degree. He or she can perform general physical examinations and take patients' medical histories. The nurse practitioner is also responsible for patient education and will often provide support to the doctors.

Research Nurse

A qualified nurse who specializes in research and whose role is to approach patients regarding possible participation in research studies. It is his or her job to supply the patient with information about the study, such as the commitment involved, the follow-up schedule, side effects, and potential complications. In some instances the research nurse is also responsible for collecting blood for the study (if it is needed) and will usually be responsible for seeing you at follow-up appointments.

PTCA Nurse

A qualified nurse, usually with several years of experience, who is responsible for overseeing the angioplasty program. Generally he or she will help to organize the angioplasty clinic lists and will oversee angioplasty referrals that have been sent from GPs, cardiologists and other hospitals. The PCTA nurse may also play a part in patient education, discharge planning, and advice. If you have a question regarding the dates and times of your angioplasty, he or she would be the person to contact.

Cath Lab Nurse

A qualified nurse who works in the cardiac catheterization laboratory. He or she may either assist the physician performing your angioplasty or help elsewhere within the cath lab. Alternatively, the cath lab nurse may work at the monitoring station or in the recovery area.

ECG Technician

A person who is specifically trained to perform ECGs on the patient. He or she may also assist in other areas that require heart monitoring, such as assisting with exercise tolerance testing or Holter tape monitoring.

Blood Technician

A person who is trained specifically to take blood, usually from the arm.

Nursing Assistant

A person who has undergone training in patient care. However, his or her training is considerably shorter than that of a registered nurse. As a result, the nursing assistant is not permitted to perform certain procedures, such as administering drugs or inserting intra-venous lines.

Medical Student

A person who is training to become a doctor.

Resident

A junior doctor in training. He or she can specialize in a particular area, such as cardiology.

Fellow

Qualified doctors, usually with a few years of experience, who are specializing in a particular area of medicine or surgery. Many fellows come from other countries to spend up to 3 years gaining additional experience.

Staff Physician

An experienced doctor who has undergone considerable training in his or her specialty and who is now in a position to make independent decisions regarding patient care and treatment. The staff physician is responsible for your overall care and for the decisions made by more junior staff.

Disclaimer: The above descriptions are intended as a general guide only. The roles of each type of staff member mentioned may differ slightly from hospital to hospital.

glossary

ACE inhibitor A drug used to treat hypertension and congestive heart failure, as well as to prevent heart attacks and worsening of angina.

Activated clotting time (ACT) A test of how much the blood has been "thinned" and how likely it is to clot.

Acute marginal branch One of the branches of the right coronary artery.

Acute myocardial infarction A heart attack.

Allen's test A test performed on the blood vessels in the wrist to check if the angioplasty can be safely performed via the radial artery in the wrist. This involves blocking the radial artery in your wrist and checking that your fingers are still receiving blood via the ulnar artery.

Anaesthetic A drug used to numb an area of skin ("local") or put someone to sleep ("general").

Aneurysm An abnormal dilatation or widening of a blood vessel due to a weakness in its wall. It can occur in a coronary artery or in a groin artery after coronary angiography or angioplasty.

Angina Chest pain caused by lack of oxygen to the heart muscle.

Angiogram *See* Angiography.

Angiography A procedure involving the injection of X-ray dye into a blood vessel and the photographing of that vessel on X-ray film. An angiogram is the still or video image produced by angiography.

Angioplasty An operation that widens narrowed blood vessels.

Anti-anginal drugs Medication used to relieve or prevent symptoms of angina.

Anticoagulant A medication that "thins" the blood by blocking the activity of proteins involved in blood clotting.

Anti-platelet drug A medication that "thins" the blood by blocking the activity of small cell fragments in the blood called platelets.

Aorta The main blood vessel of the body, which carries oxygenated blood from the heart to the rest of the body.

Aortic stenosis Narrowing of the aortic valve, resulting in increased strain on the heart muscle as it tries to pump blood through the narrowed valve. This is a cause of angina and can be corrected by valve surgery.

Aortic valve The valve through

which oxygen-rich blood leaves the heart before passing into the aorta.

Artery A blood vessel that carries oxygen-rich blood from the heart to the body tissues.

Atherosclerosis A disease that commonly narrows or blocks arteries anywhere in the body. It involves the development of a fatty, calcium-rich deposit on the inner wall of the arteries called plaque that gradually builds up over many years.

Balloon angioplasty An operation that widens narrowed blood vessels by inflating a tiny balloon inside the narrowed part of the vessel.

Beta-blocker A drug used to reduce blood pressure and/or prevent angina symptoms.

Brachial artery The artery in the elbow.

Bypass surgery *See* Coronary artery bypass graft.

CABG *See* Coronary artery bypass graft.

Calcification The hardening of tissues due to the accumulation of calcium within them.

Calcium channel blocker A drug used to reduce blood pressure and/or prevent angina symptoms.

Cardiac catheterization A procedure in which a long tube or catheter is inserted into the heart via an artery in the arm or groin. Cardiac catheterization allows physicians to carry out procedures on the heart, such as coronary angioplasty, without opening up the chest wall.

Cardiac catheterization laboratory The X-ray room where coronary angiograms and angioplasties are performed in hospitals. Also known as the "cath lab."

Cath lab *See* Cardiac catheterization laboratory.

Catheter A narrow tube that is inserted into a part of the body.

Cholesterol A type of fat that accumulates in the walls of diseased blood vessels.

Circumflex artery ("Circ") One of the three main blood vessels of the heart. It supplies oxygen to the muscle on the left side of the heart.

Clinical trial A test (of a drug or procedure) that involves patients.

Closure device A piece of equipment used to repair (close) the small hole in the artery of the leg through which an angiogram or angioplasty was performed.

Conduits The tubes used to bypass narrowed or blocked arteries during coronary bypass operations. *See also* Grafts.

Coronary angiogram

An angiogram performed on the coronary arteries.

Coronary angioplasty Angioplasty performed on the coronary arteries.

Coronary arteries The arteries that supply blood to the muscle of the heart itself. There are three main coronary arteries, the right coronary artery and the two branches of the left coronary artery.

Coronary artery bypass graft (CABG) The correct medical term for "heart bypass surgery" or "bypass surgery." This surgery is carried out to relieve angina by creating a bypass around blocked or narrowed coronary arteries. The bypass itself is a short length of artery or vein taken from the leg or chest and grafted onto the heart above and below the blocked artery.

Coronary artery disease Any disease involving the coronary arteries. Most commonly used to describe blockage of the coronary arteries due to atherosclerosis.

Cross-matching A laboratory test used to find out which type of donated blood is suitable to give a specific person for a transfusion.

Diagnostic test / procedure A test or procedure used to determine the cause of a medical disorder.

Diagonal artery One of the branches of the left anterior descending artery.

Directional atherectomy

A method of removing diseased material from narrowed blood vessels by using a cutting blade mounted on the end of a catheter.

Dissection A tear in the blood vessel wall. This can be a complication after balloon angioplasty.

Doppler flow wire A special guide wire used during angioplasty to measure the blood flow in the vessel.

Double vessel disease Heart disease involving two of the three main coronary arteries that supply the heart muscle.

Echocardiogram (Echo) An ultrasound image of the inside of the heart. Used to examine the size and function of heart structures, such as valves, and diagnose heart disorders. Usually performed by placing a transducer (probe) on the skin above the heart and is painless.

ECG *See* Electrocardiogram.

Electrocardiogram (ECG) A recording of the electrical activity of the heart. This can be useful for diagnosing angina or a heart attack.

Embolization Sudden blockage of a blood vessel due to passage of a foreign body through the blood-stream. In balloon angioplasty, it occurs when debris is released from diseased blood vessels.

Embolus A blood clot or piece of loose plaque that blocks a blood vessel.

Endothelium The normal lining of the inside of a blood vessel.

False aneurysm Not a true aneurysm (widening of a blood vessel wall), but a similar-looking swelling caused by a persistent leak in the wall. This is an occasional complication of coronary angiography or angioplasty at the point where the sheath was inserted into the groin or wrist.

General anaesthetic A drug or combination of drugs used to put a patient to sleep.

Glycoprotein IIb/IIIa inhibitors Special blood-thinning anti-platelet drugs used during angioplasty.

Graft The tube used in bypass surgery to re-route blood around blood vessel narrowings or blockages. It is usually taken from a blood vessel in the leg or chest.

Guide wire An essential piece of equipment used during every angioplasty operation. This is the first piece of equipment that is inserted along the blood vessel and across the blockage. Angioplasty equipment, such as balloons and stents, runs along the guide wire into the blood vessel.

Haematoma A bruise.

Heart attack The sudden blockage of one of the heart's blood vessels, resulting in the death of a portion of the heart muscle.

Heart bypass surgery *See* Coronary artery bypass graft.

Heart failure ("congestive" or "cardiac") The condition that results when the heart cannot, for one of a variety of reasons, pump enough blood.

Hypertension High blood pressure.

Intensive Care Unit (ICU) A specialized ward that looks after severely ill patients or those who have had major operations.

Intravascular ultrasound (IVUS) A technique that involves taking pictures of the inside of a blood vessel with probes mounted on miniaturized catheters. IVUS provides more detail than angiography.

Invasive (test) A test where part of a surgical tool enters the body.

Ischemia Lack of oxygen to the tissues. If ischemia lasts too long it can damage the tissue or even cause the tissue to die.

IVUS *See* Intravascular ultrasound.

Left anterior descending artery (LAD) One of the three main blood vessels of the heart. It supplies oxygen to the muscle at the front of the heart.

Left main coronary artery The

most important blood vessel in the heart. It divides into the left anterior descending artery and the circumflex artery.

Left main disease Disease in the left main coronary artery. In severe cases bypass surgery is usually recommended, although angioplasty may sometimes be more appropriate.

Left ventricle The main pumping chamber of the heart.

Lipid-lowering therapy Medication to lower the levels of cholesterol and other fats in the blood.

Local anaesthetic A drug that numbs the sensation of pain at the site of the injection.

Lumen The hollow space inside a blood vessel through which the blood flows.

Myocardial infarction A heart attack.

Nitrate A drug used to relieve or prevent angina symptoms.

Nitroglycerin The most commonly used nitrate drug.

Non-invasive (test) A test not requiring any equipment to be inserted into the body.

Nuclear perfusion scan A test in which a radioactive drug is injected into the body to measure the flow of blood. This test is used to diagnose angina. It can be done in addition to, or before, an angiogram.

Obtuse marginal branch (OM) One of the branches of the circumflex artery.

Occlusion A total (100 percent) blockage of a vessel.

Pacemaker The control center in the heart that determines how fast the heart beats. An artificial or temporary pacemaker is a wire that is inserted into the heart to control the heart rate.

Painless or "silent" ischemia Angina without symptoms of chest pain.

Percutaneous transluminal coronary angioplasty (PTCA) The correct medical name for angioplasty of the coronary arteries.

Pericardium The thin membrane that covers the heart.

Peripheral vascular disease (PVD) Disease that blocks the blood flow in blood vessels not in the heart (e.g., the leg arteries).

Plaque The blockage responsible for narrowing blood vessels in atherosclerosis. A plaque is usually composed of tissue cells, fatty material, and, sometimes, calcium deposits. A complicated plaque is one that has become ulcerated (broken open), contains a blood clot, or is irregular in appearance. An uncomplicated plaque is usually a smooth narrowing in a blood vessel.

Platelets Small cell fragments in the blood that are essential for blood clotting.

Positive remodelling The response of a blood vessel to the development of atherosclerosis in its wall. In the early stage of disease, the blood vessel expands in an attempt to keep the lumen of the blood vessel open and the blood flowing normally through it.

Posterior interventricular or descending branch (PIV or PDA) One of the branches of the right coronary artery. It supplies blood to the inferior surface (bottom) of the heart.

Pressure wire A special guide wire used during angioplasty to measure the blood flow in the vessel.

Prognosis A prediction of the probable outcome of a disease and how likely recovery is.

PTCA *See* Percutaneous transluminal coronary angioplasty.

Radial artery One of the two arteries in the wrist, through which angiography and angioplasty can be performed.

Radio-opaque Visible on X-rays. Radio-opaque dye is used during coronary angiography and angioplasty.

Renal failure When your kidneys do not work properly.

Re-stenosis Re-narrowing of a blood vessel that was once widened.

Revascularisation The restoration of blood flow into the heart muscle by either angioplasty or bypass surgery.

Right coronary artery (RCA) One of the three main blood vessels of the heart. It supplies oxygen to the muscle on the right side and underside of the heart.

Rotational atherectomy The removal of hard material such as calcium from narrowed or diseased blood vessels using a drill-like device. This is usually done at the same time as balloon angioplasty and stenting.

Sedative A drug that lowers the level of consciousness and makes the person feel tired or sleepy.

Sheath The short tube inserted into the blood vessel in the groin or wrist, through which longer tubes (catheters) are inserted and passed to the heart during coronary angiography or angioplasty.

Single vessel disease Heart disease involving just one of the three main blood vessels supplying the heart muscle.

Stable angina Angina that is consistently brought on by exercise or stress and does not occur during rest or sleep.

Stenosis (plural: stenoses) A blockage or narrowing of an artery.

Stent A metal coil or tube used to keep a blood vessel fully open.

Stroke Damage to the brain caused by either bleeding from a burst blood vessel in the brain or blockage by a blood clot.

Suture A stitch.

Temporary pacemaker wire A metal wire that is inserted into the heart via the leg, arm, or shoulder, to temporarily take over the heart's own pacemaker. It can be used during angioplasty if the heart rate slows down, causing a drop in blood pressure.

Thrombectomy A procedure carried out to remove a blood clot.

Thrombosis The process of blood clotting.

Thrombus (plural: thrombi) A blood clot that may block a blood vessel.

Transient ischaemic attack (TIA) A "mini-stroke" from which the person makes a full recovery.

Trans-radial approach Angioplasty performed via the wrist.

Treadmill test A test for angina during which a patient walks on a treadmill with ECG wires attached to the chest, arms, and legs.

Triple vessel disease Heart disease involving all three of the main blood vessels supplying the heart muscle.

Troponin A heart muscle protein that can be measured in a blood sample after a heart attack or episode of severe angina.

Ultrasound An imaging technique that uses sound waves.

Unstable angina Angina that develops for the first time, suddenly becomes more severe, or occurs at rest.

Vein A blood vessel that carries oxygen-poor and carbon dioxide-rich blood back to the heart and lungs.

Heart Health Information

So You're Having Heart Bypass Surgery...What Happens Next?
By Tracey Patton, Suzette Turner, and Dr. Stephen Fremes.
SCRIPT Medical Press Inc.
(to be published Spring 2002).
ISBN 0–9688982–1–1

Mended Hearts Inc.
(Canadian support available)
Support for heart disease patients.
http://www.mendedhearts.org

Heart and Stroke Foundation of Canada (Canadian)
222 Queen Street, Suite 1402
Ottawa, Ontario K1P 5V9
Tel: (613) 569-4361
Toll-free 1–888–HSF–INFO
(1–888–473–4636)
Links, news, and health tips.
www.heartandstroke.ca

Health Canada Heart Health Information (Canadian)
Links to heart health information.
http://www.hc-sc.gc.ca/english/
azindex_ghi.htm#heart

Becel Heart Health Information Bureau (Canadian)
Heart health information, recipes, and meal planning.
http://www.becelcanada.com

Heart Information Network (U.S.)
Guides on heart attacks, hypertension, heart failure, arrhythmia, and stroke, plus news, nutritional help, and general heart health information.
http://www.heartinfo.com/

Heart Disease and Cardiology Information (U.S.)
News and information on surgeries, tests, risk factors, exercise, and heart-healing devices.
http://www.heartdisease.about.com/
health/heartdisease/mbody.htm

American Heart Association (U.S.) National Center
7272 Greenville Avenue
Dallas, Texas 75231
1–800–AHA–USA1
Information on warning signs and risk factors plus a reference guide.
http://www.americanheart.org

Stress and Relaxation Information

Carleton University's Health Psychology Resources (Canadian)
Links to stress information and self-tests.
http://www.carleton.ca/~fsirois/HP_stress_links.html

Half Moon Yoga Props Ltd. (Canadian)
Find a yoga teacher near you.
http://www.halfmoonyogaprops.com/yoga_teachers.html

The Yoga Centre of Calgary (Canadian)
Yoga-related links.
http://www.yogacalgary.org/links.html

The Transcendental Meditation Program (Canada/U.S.)
Find out the benefits of, and how and where to learn, transcendental meditation.
http://www.tm.org

Sam Houston State University Counseling Center (U.S.)
Short relaxation techniques.
http://www.shsu.edu/~counsel/shortr.html

Meditation Society of America (U.S.)
Concepts and techniques of meditation plus suggested reading.
http://www.meditationsociety.com

American Yoga Association (U.S.)
General information on yoga, how to get started and how to choose a qualified yoga instructor.
http://www.americanyogaassociation.org

Nutrition and Fitness Information

Canadian Wellness (Canadian)
A directory of fitness, diet, health, nutrition, and other wellness-related professionals and their services.
http://www.canadianwellness.com

Dieticians of Canada (Canadian)
Nutrition resources and news.
http://www.dietitians.ca

Health Canada's Nutrition Resources (Canadian)
How to choose food by reading labels, Canada's Food Guide, and research reports.
http://www.hc-sc.gc.ca/hppb/nutrition/resources.htm

Canada's Physical Activity Guide (Canadian)
Guide for how to get started on an exercise program.
http://www.hc-sc.gc.ca/hppb/paguide

American Dietetic Association (U.S.)
Daily tips and features about nutrition.
http://www.eatright.org

Cookbooks

Adjey, David and Janice Holley. *Heart and Soul Cuisine: From the Estates of Sunnybrook.* Toronto: The Estates of Sunnybrook, 1997.

Moosewood Collective. *Moosewood Restaurant Favorites.* New York: Clarkson Potter, 1996.

Stern, Bonnie. *Heart Smart Cooking for Family and Friends: Great Recipes, Menus and Ideas for Casual Entertaining.* Toronto: Random House Canada, 2000.

Toronto Vegetarian Association. *Vegetarian Tastes of Toronto.* 1994

Wong, Stephen. *Heart Smart Chinese Cooking.* Vancouver: Douglas & McIntyre, 1997.

General Health Information

Telehealth Ontario
1–866–797–0000 (Canadian)
24 hours-a-day, 7 days-a-week hotline staffed by trained nurses with a least 5 years of experience. Direct links to 911 and emergency departments.

Canadian Centre for Activity and Aging (CCAA) (Canadian)
1490 Richmond Street
London, ON, N6G 2M3, Canada
Tel: (519) 661–1603
Fax: (519) 661–1612
Community information, events, research, and newsletters regarding aging.
http://www.uwo.ca/actage/index.htm

Health Canada (Canadian)
News, disease information, and links.
http://www.hc-sc.gc.ca

Canadian Health Network (Canadian)
General information about health for Canadians, including a section on heart health.
http://www.canadian-health-network.ca

HealthyWay (Canadian)
Health information from a Canadian perspective.
http://www.sympatico.ca/healthyway

HealthFinder (U.S.)
A service of the U.S. Department of Health and Human Services that connects you to publications, non-profit organizations, databases, Websites, and support groups.
http://www.healthfinder.gov

HealthAnswers (U.S.)
Health news and disease information.
http://www.healthanswers.com/home/pubHome.asp

WebMD (U.S.)
Reliable health information including news, disease and drug information, health television guide, and tips for making a personal health plan and for searching the medical library.
http://www.webmd.com

Information on Alternative Therapies

The Canadian Naturopathic Association (Canadian)
1255 Sheppard Avenue East
North York, Ontario, M2K IE2
(416) 496–8633
Toll-free automated info line:
1–877–NAT–PATH (628–7284)
General information about
naturopathic medicine.
http://www.naturopathicassoc.ca

Chinese Medicine and Acupuncture in Canada (Canadian)
Chinese medicine library, links,
success stories, and practitioners.
www.medicinechinese.com

Ontario Herbalists Association
RR#1
Port Burwell, Ontario NOJ 1T0
(416) 536-1509
Toll free: 1-877-OHA-HERB
Learn about herbalism, find out how
to participate in events, become a
member, or use helpful links.
www.herbalists.on.ca

National Center for Complementary and Alternative Medicine (U.S.)
An official source of information,
including links to other sites, current
research, and scientific information.
Tel: (301) 231–7537, ext 5
Fax: (301) 495–4957
www.nccam.nih.gov

AltMed (U.S.)
Chat, read, or ask about alternative
therapies.
http://www.altmed.com

Alternative Medicine Digest (U.S.)
What's new in alternative medicine.
http://www.alternativemedicine.com

MEDLINE Plus (U.S.)
Information on herbal remedies.
http://www.nlm.nih.gov/medlineplus/herbalmedicine.html

National Center for Homeopathy (U.S.)
801 N. Fairfax Street, Suite 306
Alexandria, Virginia 22314
Tel: (703) 548-7790
Fax: (703) 548-7792
Homeopathic resources and research
information.
http://www.homeopathic.org

American Botanical Council (U.S.)
P.O. Box 144345
Austin, Texas
78714-4345
abc@herbalgram.org
Research, links, science-based information on herbs and phytomedicines.
http://www.herbalgram.org

your diary

Contact Information

Name of Current Family Doctor	Address	Phone	Fax	Email
Hospital	Address	Phone	Fax	Email
Name of Current Doctor (specialist)	Address	Phone	Fax	Email
Name of Angioplasty Nurse	Address	Phone	Fax	Email

Clinic Visits

Date	Time	Address	Doctor	Purpose

Date	Time	Address	Doctor	Purpose

Test Results

Test	Date	Doctor	Purpose	Results

Test	Date	Doctor	Purpose	Results

Current and Past Medications (including complementary therapies and supplements)

Drug Name	Date Began Drug	Purpose of Drug	Dosage	Side Effects	Dosage Instructions

Drug Name	Date Began Drug	Purpose of Drug	Dosage	Side Effects	Dosage Instructions

Symptoms

Symptom	Date	Time	Cause	Severity on Scale of 1 to 10 (1=mild, 10=severe)	Duration

Symptom	Date	Time	Cause	Severity on Scale of 1 to 10 (1=mild, 10=severe)	Duration

Questions for the Doctor

About the surgery:

About the kind of transportation I should arrange for the day before and after the surgery:

About what I should wear the day of the surgery:

About what will happen before the surgery:

About what will happen after the surgery:

About what I should do to help my recovery (diet, exercise, supervision):

About what my physical limitations will be after surgery:

Rehabilitation Clinic/Other Wellness Center Contact Information

Address	Phone	Fax	Email

My Lifestyle Goals: Current Weight _____

Notes

Notes

index

References to figures: *3fig*;
references to tables: *119t*;
references to More Detail boxes in bold: **4**;
references to Key Point boxes in bold italic: ***5***;
references to Self-Help boxes in italic: *12*